NOURISHING

DIET PLAN

FOR

ANTI INFLAMMATION

Essential Healing Foods to Take Back Your Health

TABLE OF CONTENT

INTRODUCTION

Our bodies often struggle with silent inflammation, a quiet adversary that gradually erodes our health from the inside out in a world full of environmental pollutants, highly processed foods, and chronic stress. Although inflammation is a normal reaction to damage or infection, it may become uncontrollably high when it is brought on by unhealthful eating habits, which can result in a variety of chronic illnesses including diabetes, cancer, arthritis, and heart disease. But what if the basic, natural foods we eat on a daily basis hold the secret to regaining your health and vigor instead of the newest pharmaceutical discovery?

More than simply a manual, **Nourishing Diet Plan for Anti-Inflammation: Essential Healing Foods to Reclaim Your Health** is a road map for improving both your connection with food and your overall health. This book provides a thorough and useful guide to internal healing as it examines the intriguing relationship between the foods we consume and our bodies' inflammatory reactions. You may bring your body back into balance, lessen inflammation, and regain the bright health that is naturally yours by embracing the healing power of nature's abundance.

During this journey, you will learn how to feed your body with tasty anti-inflammatory foods that also support your body's natural healing processes. You'll discover how to recognize and cut out the items in your diet that cause inflammation, swapping them out with nutrient-dense, healing meals. This book offers the information, techniques, and recipes you need to regain control over your health, whether you're coping with a chronic illness, trying to avoid illness, or just wanting to feel your best.

These pages contain:

- Science-backed insights on the relationship between certain foods and inflammation as well as general health.
- Detailed meal plans and recipes developed to minimize inflammation and promote recovery.
- Useful advice for cooking and leading an anti-inflammatory lifestyle.

The path to wellness is fundamentally universal yet very individualized. By the time you finish reading this book, you will have the ability to make decisions that promote both the short- and long-term health of your body. Your diet has the potential to be your most effective weapon against inflammation and contribute to a longer, healthier, and more energetic life.

1: Why, How and For Who?

The Science behind Inflammation

Inflammation is a complex biological response of body tissues to harmful stimuli, such as pathogens, damaged cells, or irritants. It is a protective response that involves immune cells, blood vessels, and molecular mediators. The purpose of inflammation is essentially to eliminate the initial cause of cell injury, clear out damaged cells and tissues, and initiate tissue repair.

Key aspects of inflammation's purpose include:

a) Protection: Inflammation helps isolate and contain the damaged area, preventing the spread of infection or injury to nearby tissues.

b) Clearance: It facilitates the removal of pathogens, damaged cells, and debris from the affected area.

c) Healing: Inflammation initiates the healing process by promoting tissue repair and regeneration.

d) Adaptation: It can help the body adapt to stress or changes in the environment.

The classic signs of inflammation, first described by Celsus in the 1st century AD, are:

- Rubor (redness): Due to increased blood flow to the affected area
- Calor (heat): Also resulting from increased blood flow
- Tumor (swelling): Caused by fluid accumulation in tissues
- Dolor (pain): Due to the release of chemicals that stimulate nerve endings

- Functio laesa (loss of function): Added later by Galen, referring to the impaired function of the inflamed area

It's important to note that inflammation is not inherently harmful. In fact, it's a crucial part of the body's defense mechanism. However, when inflammation becomes chronic or occurs in the wrong context, it can contribute to various diseases and disorders.

Inflammation can occur in response to a wide range of stimuli, including:

1. Physical injuries (cuts, burns, etc.)
2. Infections (bacterial, viral, fungal)
3. Chemical irritants
4. Radiation exposure
5. Autoimmune reactions
6. Chronic stress

Types of Inflammation (Acute vs. Chronic)

Inflammation is typically categorized into two main types: acute and chronic. These differ in their duration, cause, and overall impact on the body.

a) Acute Inflammation:

Acute inflammation is the body's initial response to harmful stimuli. It typically lasts for a short period, from a few hours to a few days.

Characteristics of acute inflammation include:
- Rapid onset
- Short duration (usually resolves within days or weeks)
- Primarily mediated by neutrophils (a type of white blood cell)
- Usually results in resolution and healing

Examples of conditions involving acute inflammation:
- Acute bronchitis
- Cuts and scrapes
- Acute appendicitis
- Tonsillitis

- Acute sinusitis

b) Chronic Inflammation:

Chronic inflammation is a prolonged, dysregulated response that can last for months or even years. It can result from failure to eliminate the cause of acute inflammation, persistent exposure to a low-level irritant, or autoimmune disorders.

Characteristics of chronic inflammation include:
- Slower onset
- Long duration (weeks, months, or years)
- Primarily mediated by mononuclear cells (lymphocytes and macrophages)
- Simultaneous destruction and healing of tissue

Examples of conditions involving chronic inflammation:
- Rheumatoid arthritis
- Atherosclerosis
- Chronic obstructive pulmonary disease (COPD)
- Inflammatory bowel diseases (e.g., Crohn's disease, ulcerative colitis)
- Some cancers

Key differences between acute and chronic inflammation:

1. Duration: Acute is short-term, while chronic is long-term.
2. Cell types involved: Acute primarily involves neutrophils, while chronic involves lymphocytes and macrophages.
3. Outcome: Acute often leads to resolution, while chronic can lead to tissue damage and disease.
4. Systemic effects: Chronic inflammation often has more significant systemic effects on the body.

Understood. Let's move on to the inflammatory response process.

The Inflammatory Response Process

The inflammatory response is a complex, coordinated sequence of events that occurs when the body encounters harmful stimuli. This process involves various cells, tissues, and chemical mediators.

a) Recognition of Threat:
- Cells in the affected area (e.g., tissue-resident macrophages) detect the presence of pathogens or tissue damage through pattern recognition receptors (PRRs).
- These receptors recognize pathogen-associated molecular patterns (PAMPs) or damage-associated molecular patterns (DAMPs).

b) Initiation of Response:
- Activated cells release inflammatory mediators such as histamine, prostaglandins, and cytokines.
- These mediators cause local blood vessels to dilate (vasodilation) and become more permeable.

c) Vascular Changes:
- Increased blood flow to the area (causing redness and heat).
- Increased vascular permeability allows plasma proteins and leukocytes to move into the tissue.

d) Cellular Events:
- Leukocytes (primarily neutrophils in acute inflammation) are recruited to the site.
- These cells adhere to the blood vessel walls and migrate into the tissue (a process called extravasation).

e) Phagocytosis and Pathogen Elimination:
- Neutrophils and macrophages engulf and destroy pathogens and cellular debris through phagocytosis.
- They also release antimicrobial substances and reactive oxygen species.

f) Release of Inflammatory Mediators:
- Activated immune cells release additional cytokines and chemokines.
- These further amplify the inflammatory response and recruit more immune cells.

g) Resolution and Repair:

- As the threat is neutralized, anti-inflammatory mediators are produced.
- These help to resolve inflammation and initiate tissue repair.
- Specialized pro-resolving mediators (SPMs) play a crucial role in this phase.

h) Tissue Remodeling:
- Damaged tissue is repaired or replaced.
- This may involve the formation of scar tissue in some cases.

Throughout this process, various feedback mechanisms regulate the intensity and duration of the inflammatory response. Dysregulation at any stage can lead to excessive or prolonged inflammation, potentially causing tissue damage or chronic inflammatory conditions.

It's worth noting that while this general process applies to most instances of inflammation, the specific details can vary depending on the type of tissue involved and the nature of the inflammatory stimulus.

Symptoms and Signs of Inflammation

Inflammation can manifest in various ways, depending on its location, cause, and severity. The classic signs of inflammation, first described by Celsus in the 1st century AD, are still relevant today. These are often accompanied by additional symptoms.

a) Classical Signs of Inflammation (Latin terms):

1. Rubor (Redness):
- Due to increased blood flow to the affected area
- More noticeable in superficial inflammations

2. Calor (Heat):
- Also resulting from increased blood flow
- Can be detected by touch or thermal imaging

3. Tumor (Swelling):
- Caused by fluid accumulation (edema) in tissues
- Can lead to pressure on nerve endings, contributing to pain

4. Dolor (Pain):
- Due to the release of chemicals that stimulate nerve endings
- Can range from mild discomfort to severe pain

5. Functio laesa (Loss of function):
- Added later by Galen
- Refers to impaired function of the inflamed area

b) Additional Symptoms and Signs:

1. Systemic symptoms:
- Fever: Caused by pyrogens acting on the hypothalamus
- Fatigue: Common in both acute and chronic inflammation
- Malaise: General feeling of discomfort or illness

2. Localized symptoms:
- Stiffness: Especially in joint inflammation
- Itching: Can occur in certain types of inflammation, particularly skin conditions

3. Organ-specific symptoms:
- Respiratory: Cough, shortness of breath (in lung inflammation)
- Gastrointestinal: Nausea, vomiting, diarrhea (in gut inflammation)
- Neurological: Headache, confusion (in brain inflammation)

4. Laboratory findings:
- Elevated white blood cell count (leukocytosis)
- Increased levels of acute phase proteins (e.g., C-reactive protein)
- Elevated erythrocyte sedimentation rate (ESR)

5. Imaging findings:
- Increased uptake on PET scans
- Contrast enhancement on MRI or CT scans
- Increased blood flow on Doppler ultrasound

c) Chronic Inflammation Symptoms:

- Often more subtle than acute inflammation
- May include persistent fatigue, body pain, mood disorders, gastrointestinal issues
- Can lead to weight changes, sleep disturbances, and frequent infections

d) Variability in Presentation:
- Symptoms can vary greatly depending on the affected tissue or organ
- Some inflammations may be "silent" with few overt symptoms
- Severity can range from mild to life-threatening

These symptoms are essential for identifying inflammatory diseases and tracking their development or improvement. Nevertheless, it should be mentioned that these indicators may not always indicate the level of inflammation, particularly in cases when the inflammation is persistent or deeply rooted.

Causes of Inflammation

Inflammation can be triggered by a wide variety of factors. Understanding these causes is crucial for both prevention and treatment of inflammatory conditions. Here are the main categories of inflammation causes:

a) Pathogens:
1. Bacteria: Both extracellular and intracellular bacteria
2. Viruses: Including influenza, coronavirus, HIV
3. Fungi: Such as Candida species
4. Parasites: Like malaria or toxoplasma

b) Physical Injuries:
1. Trauma: Cuts, bruises, fractures
2. Burns: Thermal, chemical, or radiation burns
3. Frostbite
4. Foreign bodies: Splinters, shrapnel

c) Chemical Irritants:
1. Toxins: Both endogenous and exogenous
2. Alcohol

3. Cigarette smoke
4. Environmental pollutants

d) Radiation:
1. UV radiation from sunlight
2. Ionizing radiation (X-rays, gamma rays)

e) Autoimmune Disorders:
1. Rheumatoid arthritis
2. Systemic lupus erythematosus
3. Multiple sclerosis
4. Type 1 diabetes

f) Allergic Reactions:
1. Food allergies
2. Drug allergies
3. Environmental allergies (pollen, dust mites)

g) Chronic Stress:
1. Psychological stress
2. Physical stress (e.g., lack of sleep, overexertion)

h) Obesity:
- Adipose tissue produces pro-inflammatory cytokines

i) Dietary Factors:
1. High intake of saturated fats
2. Excessive sugar consumption
3. Processed foods

j) Genetic Factors:
- Certain genetic mutations can predispose to inflammatory conditions

k) Age-related Changes:
- Inflammaging": Low-grade chronic inflammation associated with aging

l) Environmental Factors:

1. Pollution
2. Extreme temperatures
3. High altitudes

m) Tissue Necrosis:
- Cell death due to injury or disease can trigger inflammation

n) Ischemia:
- Lack of blood supply leading to tissue damage

o) Mechanical Stress:
1. Repetitive motion injuries
2. Pressure ulcers

p) Hormonal Changes:
- Can influence inflammatory responses, particularly in autoimmune conditions

q) Gut Dysbiosis:
- Imbalance in gut microbiota can lead to systemic inflammation

Not only that, but inflammation is usually induced by more than one of these variables working together. An unhealthy diet or high levels of stress, for instance, might make a bacterial illness worse. On top of that, inflammation may become a vicious cycle when it persists for an extended period of time.

It is essential to identify the root cause of inflammation in order to formulate effective treatment plans. Resolving inflammation may be as simple as eliminating the irritant or curing an infection, depending on the situation. On the other hand, a more nuanced and multi-pronged strategy can be required when dealing with chronic inflammation.

Recap

Inflammation is the body's way of protecting itself and starting the healing process. It's like the body's alarm system that goes off when something's wrong.

There are two main types:

1. Short-term (acute) inflammation: This is like a quick response team. It happens fast and usually goes away once the problem is fixed.

2. Long-term (chronic) inflammation: This is when the alarm keeps ringing even after the initial problem is gone. It's like the body is stuck in defense mode.

When inflammation happens, you might notice:
- Redness
- Swelling
- Heat
- Pain
- Difficulty using the affected area normally

Inflammation can be caused by lots of things, like:
- Injuries (cuts, burns, etc.)
- Germs (bacteria, viruses)
- Allergies
- Stress
- Poor diet
- Being overweight

Your immune system is the main player in inflammation. It sends out special cells to fight off invaders or heal damage. These cells release chemicals that cause the signs of inflammation we can see and feel.

While short-term inflammation is helpful, long-term inflammation can lead to serious health problems. It's linked to many common diseases like:
- Heart disease
- Diabetes
- Arthritis
- Some types of cancer
- Alzheimer's disease

To fight inflammation, doctors might recommend:
- Medicines like ibuprofen or stronger prescription drugs
- Changes in diet (eating more fruits, vegetables, and fish)

- Regular exercise
- Stress reduction techniques like meditation
- Getting enough sleep

Researchers are always looking for new ways to control inflammation and treat the diseases it causes. They're especially interested in finding ways to stop long-term inflammation without shutting down the body's ability to protect itself.

Who Should Eat Inflammation Healing Foods

1. People with Chronic Inflammatory Conditions: Individuals diagnosed with chronic inflammatory diseases should prioritize anti-inflammatory foods in their diet. These conditions include:

a) Rheumatoid Arthritis
b) Inflammatory Bowel Disease (Crohn's Disease, Ulcerative Colitis)
c) Psoriasis and Psoriatic Arthritis
d) Systemic Lupus Erythematosus
e) Multiple Sclerosis
f) Ankylosing Spondylitis

For these individuals, an anti-inflammatory diet can help manage symptoms, reduce flare-ups, and potentially slow disease progression. It's important to note that while diet can be a powerful tool, it should be used in conjunction with, not as a replacement for, prescribed medical treatments.

2. People with Autoimmune Disorders: Many autoimmune disorders involve chronic inflammation. People with conditions such as:

a) Hashimoto's Thyroiditis
b) Type 1 Diabetes
c) Celiac Disease
d) Graves' Disease

May benefit from incorporating anti-inflammatory foods into their diet. These foods can help modulate the immune response and potentially reduce the severity of symptoms.

3. Individuals with Cardiovascular Disease: Inflammation plays a crucial role in the development and progression of cardiovascular diseases. People with or at risk for the following conditions should consider an anti-inflammatory diet:

a) Atherosclerosis
b) Coronary Artery Disease
c) Hypertension
d) History of Heart Attack or Stroke

Anti-inflammatory foods, particularly those rich in omega-3 fatty acids, can help improve heart health and reduce the risk of cardiovascular events.

4. People with Metabolic Disorders: Chronic low-grade inflammation is often associated with metabolic disorders. Individuals with the following conditions may benefit from anti-inflammatory foods:

a) Type 2 Diabetes
b) Metabolic Syndrome
c) Obesity
d) Non-Alcoholic Fatty Liver Disease (NAFLD)

An anti-inflammatory diet can help improve insulin sensitivity, promote weight loss, and reduce the risk of complications associated with these conditions.

5. Individuals with Chronic Pain: Many chronic pain conditions have an inflammatory component. People suffering from:

a) Fibromyalgia
b) Chronic Back Pain
c) Osteoarthritis
d) Chronic Headaches or Migraines

May find relief by incorporating anti-inflammatory foods into their diet. These foods can help reduce pain and improve overall quality of life.

6. People with Allergies and Asthma: Allergic reactions and asthma involve inflammatory processes. Individuals with these conditions may benefit from anti-inflammatory foods to help manage symptoms and reduce the frequency of flare-ups.

7. Those with Skin Conditions: Many skin conditions have an inflammatory component. People with the following may benefit from an anti-inflammatory diet:

a) Acne
b) Eczema
c) Rosacea

8. Older Adults: As we age, our bodies tend to experience more chronic, low-grade inflammation, a phenomenon known as "inflammaging." Older adults can potentially slow down age-related decline and improve overall health by consuming anti-inflammatory foods.

9. Athletes and Physically Active Individuals: Intense physical activity can lead to acute inflammation. Athletes and those who exercise regularly can benefit from anti-inflammatory foods to aid in recovery and reduce exercise-induced inflammation.

10. People under Chronic Stress: Chronic stress can lead to systemic inflammation. Individuals experiencing ongoing stress from work, personal life, or other sources may find that anti-inflammatory foods help mitigate the physical effects of stress.

11. Smokers and Ex-smokers: Smoking causes significant inflammation in the body. Current smokers and those who have recently quit can potentially reduce smoking-related inflammation by focusing on anti-inflammatory foods.

12. People Exposed to Environmental Toxins: Individuals who live in areas with high pollution or who are regularly exposed to environmental toxins may benefit from the protective effects of anti-inflammatory foods.

13. Anyone Interested in Preventive Health: Even if you don't have a specific health condition, incorporating anti-inflammatory foods into your diet can be beneficial for overall health and disease prevention. These foods are generally nutrient-dense and support overall well-being.

Keep in mind that the point of eating anti-inflammatory foods is to promote health and wellness in general, not only to lower inflammation. In general, these foods are beneficial for almost everyone's health since they are part of a balanced, nutritious diet.

Therapeutic Lifestyle Practices for Inflammatory Relief

I can attest from personal experience that therapeutic lifestyle practices are crucial for symptom management and general quality of life improvement while dealing with chronic inflammation, which I have endured for many years. As someone who has struggled with stress, poor sleep hygiene, and a lack of control over their chronic health, I would like to share my story and the methods that have helped me the most in these three areas. Other people may find value in my story if they are going through the same things I have.

Stress Management Techniques:

One of the main things that has usually set off my inflammatory flare-ups is stress. I've accumulated a toolbox of stress-reduction strategies throughout time, and they've really improved my life.

My everyday routine now revolves on mindfulness meditation. Every morning, I begin with a 15-minute practice led by apps like Calm or Headspace. Calming my thoughts was difficult for me at first, but with practice, it's become easier. I've found that when I meditate, I'm better able to deal with stresses when they come up.

For me, deep breathing exercises have also changed the game. I take a few minutes to practice box breathing whenever I feel my stress level rising throughout the day. I inhale for four counts, hold my breath for four, release my breath for four, and then repeat the process for four more times. This easy method helps me concentrate and refresh, which often stops stress from becoming worse.

Another thing that has helped me a lot is journaling. I take ten minutes every evening to write down my problems, thoughts, and things for which I am thankful. I can better manage my emotions and put my worries in perspective when I engage in this activity. It helps me to release my anger outside instead of allowing them to fester within while I'm experiencing pain or other symptoms.

Reconnecting with nature has also shown to be an effective way to reduce stress. Whether it's strolling at a local park or just lounging in my garden, I make it a point to spend at least half an hour outdoors every day. My body and mind appear to be soothed by the mix of mild activity, fresh air, and beautiful surroundings.

Good Sleep Hygiene:

My ability to control my inflammation has greatly improved since I changed my sleeping patterns. I have finally figured out a sleep schedule that works for me, but it took some trial and error.

I started by establishing a regular sleep regimen. Every day, including weekends, I go to bed and get up at the same hour. My body's natural clock has been regulated as a result, which has made it simpler for me to go to sleep and get up.

I've established a calming nighttime ritual that lets my body know when it's time to unwind. I turn down the lights in my home and stay away from any electronics around an hour before bed. My favorite way to relax is to take a warm bath with Epsom salts; it helps with joint pain and soothes my thoughts.

My bedroom is now a haven for rest. I made an investment in supportive pillows and a cozy mattress. I maintain the room silent, dark, and cold. To drown out any annoying noises, I use white noise machines and blackout drapes.

I pay attention to what I eat at night. I try to stay away from coffee after 2:00 PM and avoid eating large meals just before bed. I've discovered that unwinding with a cup of chamomile tea an hour before bed is beneficial.

If, after 20 minutes, I still can't go back to sleep after waking up in the middle of the night, I get up and read a book or anything peaceful instead of using a screen till I feel drowsy again. This keeps me from becoming irritated and lying in bed, which may make it much more difficult to fall asleep.

Exercise Routine for Chronic Ailments:

It has been essential to create a fitness regimen that complements rather than contradicts my chronic illness. I've discovered that striking a balance between maintaining an active lifestyle and not overdoing it is crucial.

My workout regimen now consists mostly of low-impact exercises. Swimming has been very advantageous. Because the water's buoyancy relieves strain on my joints, I can exercise effectively without aggravating my problems. I aim to go swimming three times a week for thirty minutes.

For me, somatic movements have also had a transformational effect. I engage in somatic exercises, emphasizing deep stretches and deliberate, slow motions. This has relieved tension and helped me become more strong and flexible. Twice a week, I go to class, and on the other days, I work out briefly at home.

Another important part of my regimen is walking. When I'm feeling well, I try to go for a stroll for thirty minutes. I may only be able to move for 10 minutes at a time when my symptoms flare-up, but even this little bit of mobility may help.

For the purpose of preserving bone density and muscle mass, strength training has proved crucial. My physical therapist has assisted me in creating a regimen that incorporates resistance bands and small weights. Our main emphasis is on workouts that minimize the strain on my joints.

I've discovered that I can listen to my body and modify my workout schedule as necessary. I may do a little bit more on good days and less on bad. Rather than intensity, consistency has proven to be the key.

I also include active recuperation in my daily regimen. This may be taking a leisurely stroll, using a foam roller, or doing some light stretching. I can maintain my mobility with these exercises without overtaxing my body.

There have been difficulties and obstacles in putting these lifestyle patterns into effect. But taking care of my stress, getting better sleep, and sticking to a regular exercise schedule has all added up to greatly lowering my inflammation and enhancing my general wellbeing.

I now understand that recovery is a nonlinear process. Even though I have good and terrible days, having these routines in place makes it easier for me to deal with the difficulties. Having the skills to actively manage my health gives me a sense of empowerment.

I urge you to look into these options if you're struggling with persistent inflammation and see what suits you the best. Always practice self-compassion and acknowledge your little accomplishments as you progress. As I have discovered, these lifestyle choices may significantly reduce inflammation and enhance your quality of life with enough time and effort.

Stress Management Techniques

1. Mindfulness and Meditation: Practicing mindfulness and meditation can help calm the mind and reduce stress. Techniques such as focused breathing, body scans, and guided imagery can be particularly effective.
2. Physical Activity: Exercise is a powerful stress reliever. Activities like walking, running, yoga, and tai chi can help reduce stress hormones and increase endorphins, which improve mood.
3. Deep Breathing Exercises: Deep breathing helps activate the body's relaxation response. Techniques like diaphragmatic breathing and the 4-7-8 method can be practiced anywhere to quickly reduce stress.
4. Support System: Connecting with friends and family can provide emotional support and reduce feelings of stress. Talking about your feelings and experiences can help you feel understood and less isolated.
5. Hobbies and Leisure Activities: Engaging in activities you enjoy, such as reading, gardening, or playing a musical instrument, can provide a mental break and reduce stress levels.

Good Sleep Hygiene

Good sleep hygiene involves practices that promote consistent, quality sleep.

1. Maintain a Consistent Sleep Schedule: Go to bed and wake up at the same time every day, even on weekends. This helps regulate your body's internal clock and improves sleep quality.
2. Create a Relaxing Bedtime Routine: Develop a pre-sleep routine that helps you unwind. This could include activities like reading, taking a warm bath, or practicing relaxation exercises.
3. Optimize Your Sleep Environment: Ensure your bedroom is conducive to sleep. Keep it cool, dark, and quiet. Consider using blackout curtains, earplugs, or a white noise machine if needed.
4. Limit Exposure to Screens before Bed: The blue light emitted by phones, tablets, and computers can interfere with your sleep. Try to avoid screens at least an hour before bedtime.
5. Be Mindful of Food and Drink: Avoid large meals, caffeine, and alcohol close to bedtime. These can disrupt your sleep cycle and reduce sleep quality.

Exercise Routine for Chronic Ailments

Regular exercise is crucial for managing chronic ailments. Here are some guidelines for creating an exercise routine:

1. Start slowly and Build Up: If you're new to exercise or have been inactive, start with low-impact activities like walking or swimming. Gradually increase the intensity and duration as your fitness improves.
2. Include a Variety of Exercises
- Incorporate different types of exercises to address various aspects of fitness
- Aerobic Exercise: Activities like walking, cycling, and swimming improve cardiovascular health.
- Strength Training: Use weights or resistance bands to build muscle strength and support joint health.
- Flexibility Exercises: Stretching and yoga can improve flexibility and reduce stiffness.

3. Listen to Your Body: Pay attention to how your body responds to exercise. If you experience pain or discomfort, adjust your routine accordingly. It's important to find a balance that allows you to stay active without exacerbating your condition.

4. Stay Consistent: Consistency is key to reaping the benefits of exercise. Aim for at least 150 minutes of moderate-intensity exercise per week, spread across several days.

Elimination Diet Plan

An organized eating regimen called the Elimination Diet is intended to help identify things that may be generating negative responses in the body. The diet consists of two primary stages: the period of elimination and the phase of reintroduction.

1. The Elimination Phase:

The foundation of this nutritional strategy is the elimination phase. You cut out potentially toxic foods from your diet during this phase for a certain amount of time, usually two to four weeks. This stage calls for dedication and thorough preparation.

Key aspects of the elimination phase:

a) Foods to Eliminate:
The most common foods eliminated include:
- Dairy products
- Gluten-containing grains (wheat, barley, rye)
- Soy
- Eggs
- Nuts and seeds
- Nightshade vegetables (tomatoes, peppers, eggplant, potatoes)
- Citrus fruits
- Shellfish
- Corn
- Pork
- Beef
- Coffee
- Alcohol
- Processed foods and artificial additives

b) Duration: Usually, the elimination phase lasts two to four weeks. This length of time gives your body adequate time to rid itself of any possible allergens or irritants and for your symptoms to become better.

c) Meal Planning: During this phase, your diet will primarily consist of:
- Fruits (except citrus)
- Most vegetables (except nightshades)
- Lean meats like chicken and turkey
- Fish (except shellfish)
- Rice and quinoa
- Healthy fats like olive oil and avocado

d) Keeping a Food Journal: During this time, keeping a thorough diet log is essential. Keep track of everything you consume as well as any symptoms you encounter. As you advance, this will help you see trends and areas for improvement.

e) Reading Labels: Read food labels carefully to make sure you're not unintentionally ingesting anything that has been banned. Many processed foods have hidden additives.

f) Preparation: Before starting the elimination phase, it's advisable to:
- Clear your pantry of eliminated foods
- Plan your meals in advance
- Stock up on allowed foods
- Inform family and friends about your dietary changes for support

g) Potential Challenges:
- Initial discomfort or cravings as your body adjusts
- Difficulty eating out or in social situations
- Possible temporary worsening of symptoms (known as a "healing crisis")

h) Monitoring Progress: Be mindful of your feelings throughout this stage. Numerous individuals claim increases in their general well-being, energy levels, digestion, and skin clarity.

2. The Reintroduction Phase:

The period of reintroduction has similar significance and requires meticulous implementation. This stage assists in determining whether particular meals could be problematic.

Key aspects of the reintroduction phase:

a) Timing: Only when you've finished the whole elimination phase and your symptoms have considerably improved, should you start the reintroduction phase.

b) Systematic Approach: Reintroduce foods one by one, in a predetermined sequence. Move on to meals that are more often troublesome after starting with those that are least likely to produce responses.

c) Process for Each Food:
- Choose one food to reintroduce
- Eat a small amount of this food on day one
- Increase the amount slightly on day two
- On day three, eat a normal portion of this food
- Observe and record any symptoms for the next 2-3 days
- If no reactions occur, keep this food in your diet and move on to the next food
- If you experience a reaction, remove the food and wait until symptoms subside before trying the next food

d) Reintroduction Schedule: A typical reintroduction schedule might look like this:
Week 1: Dairy (start with yogurt, then milk, then cheese)
Week 2: Eggs
Week 3: Gluten-free grains (oats, corn)
Week 4: Gluten-containing grains
Week 5: Soy
Week 6: Nuts and seeds
Week 7: Nightshade vegetables
... And so on

e) Detailed Symptom Tracking: During reintroduction, it's crucial to track symptoms meticulously. Look for:
- Digestive issues (bloating, gas, diarrhea, constipation)
- Skin reactions (rashes, acne, itching)

- Headaches or migraines
- Fatigue or energy changes
- Mood swings
- Joint pain
- Sleep disturbances
- Any other unusual symptoms

f) Interpreting Results:
- Immediate reactions (within hours) are easier to identify
- Delayed reactions can occur up to 72 hours after consuming a food
- Some reactions might be dose-dependent (only occurring with larger amounts)

g) Challenges in Reintroduction:
- Patience is key; the process can take several weeks or even months
- It can be tempting to reintroduce foods too quickly
- Distinguishing between food reactions and other factors (stress, illness) can be difficult

h) After Reintroduction: Once you've completed the reintroduction phase:
- You'll have a clearer picture of which foods you tolerate well and which cause issues
- Create a personalized diet plan based on your findings

i) Long-term Approach:
- Some people may need to permanently avoid certain trigger foods
- Others might be able to reintroduce problematic foods in small amounts or on an occasional basis
- Periodic "elimination breaks" can be helpful for managing symptoms long-term

Important Considerations:

1. Medical Supervision: An elimination diet should always be followed under a doctor's supervision, particularly if you have any underlying medical illnesses or dietary issues.
2. Nutritional Balance: Make sure you're consuming enough food while going through the elimination stage. Creating a balanced food plan might be assisted by a dietician.

3. Food Allergies vs. Intolerances: Rather than treating actual allergies, this diet is more suited for determining food sensitivities or intolerances. Management of severe allergies must be distinct.
4. Psychological Aspect: Recognize the possible psychological effects of rigid diets. All the while, I have a positive connection with food.
5. Not a Long-term Diet: The elimination diet is not a long-term eating regimen; rather, it is a diagnostic tool. Finding foods that cause problems and designing a balanced, sustainable diet that suits your needs are the main objectives.
6. Individual Variations: Everybody will react differently to the elimination diet. A person's symptoms may not be triggered in another.

The Elimination Diet Plan may be an effective strategy for determining dietary sensitivities and enhancing general health, especially when it comes to the elimination and reintroduction stages. But it takes dedication, perseverance, and meticulous execution. When carried out properly, it may provide insightful information on the effects of various foods on your body, empowering you to make wise long-term dietary decisions.

CHAPTER 2

SMOOTHIES AND DRINKS

Berry Banana Smoothie

Mango Ginger Smoothie

Turmeric Pineapple Smoothie

Apple Spinach Smoothie

Beetroot Berry Smoothie

Cherry Almond Smoothie

Citrus Carrot Smoothie

Blueberry Avocado Smoothie

Green Smoothie

Strawberry Basil Smoothie

Ginger Peach Smoothie

Cucumber Mint Smoothie

Papaya Turmeric Smoothie

Raspberry Chia Smoothie

Pomegranate Beet Smoothie

Kiwi Spinach Smoothie

Orange Carrot Smoothie

Watermelon Mint Smoothie

Apple Cinnamon Smoothie

Berry Banana Smoothie

Calories per Serving:
200

Prep Time: 5 minutes Serving Size: 2 servings

Fat: 4g

Protein: 6g

Carbs: 34g

1 cup frozen mixed berries	1/2 cup water or more
1 ripe banana, peeled and sliced	1 tablespoon almond butter
1/2 cup frozen cauliflower florets	1/2 teaspoon cinnamon
1 tablespoon chia seeds	
1/2 teaspoon ground turmeric	
1 cup unsweetened almond milk	

Gluten-Free: Yes

Dairy-Free: Yes

Vegan: Yes

Nut-Free: Yes

1. Get everything you need, and make sure the cauliflower and banana are frozen. Smoothies made using frozen ingredients have a thicker and creamier consistency
2. Add the frozen mixed berries, banana slices, frozen cauliflower, chia seeds, turmeric, almond milk, and water to a high-speed blender. Combine almond butter and cinnamon at this point if using.
3. Begin with a low speed and gradually raise it to high as the blender starts to run. Scrape down the sides of the blender as required to get a smooth smoothie. Blend until smooth. Just add extra water until the smoothie reaches the consistency you want if it's too thick.
4. Two glasses should be filled with the smoothie.

For more protein, you may add a scoop of plant-based protein powder.

Mango Ginger Smoothie

**Calories per Serving:
180**

Fat: 3g

Protein: 3g

Carbs: 39g

Prep Time: 5 minutes Serving Size: 2 servings

1 1/2 cups frozen mango chunks

1/2 inch fresh ginger, peeled and grated or 1/2 teaspoon ground ginger.

1/2 banana, peeled and sliced

1/2 cup coconut water or plain water

1 cup unsweetened coconut milk

1 tablespoon ground flaxseed

1/2 teaspoon turmeric

1/2 teaspoon lime juice

Gluten-Free: Yes

Dairy-Free: Yes

Vegan: Yes

Nut-Free: Yes

1. Gather all the components. Ensure the mango chunks are frozen to make a thick, delicious smoothie.
2. Add the frozen mango chunks, grated fresh ginger, banana slices, coconut water, and coconut milk to a high-speed blender. If using, add the ground flaxseed, turmeric, and lime juice.
3. Begin with a low speed and gradually raise it to high as the blender starts to run. Scrape down the sides of the blender as required to get a smooth smoothie. Blend until smooth. Adjust the consistency by adding additional coconut water if required.
4. Two glasses should be filled with the smoothie.

For added creaminess, you may add a tiny quantity of avocado, which also delivers healthy fats.

Turmeric Pineapple Smoothie

Calories per Serving: 160

Fat: 3g

Protein: 2g

Carbs: 35g

Prep Time: 5 minutes Serving Size: 2 servings

1 1/2 cups frozen pineapple chunks

1/2 teaspoon ground turmeric or 1/2 inch fresh turmeric root, peeled and grated

1/2 banana, peeled and sliced

1/2 cup coconut water

1 cup unsweetened almond milk

1/2 teaspoon ground ginger or 1/2 inch fresh ginger, peeled and grated.

1 tablespoon chia seeds

1/2 teaspoon ground cinnamon

A pinch of black pepper

Gluten-Free: Yes

Dairy-Free: Yes

Vegan: Yes

Nut-Free: Yes

1. Gather all the ingredients and make sure the pineapple is frozen for a thick, chilly smoothie.
2. Add the frozen pineapple chunks, turmeric, banana slices, coconut water, and almond milk to a high-speed blender. If using, add the ginger, chia seeds, cinnamon, and a sprinkle of black pepper.
3. Start blending on low speed, then gradually raise to high. Blend until the smoothie is smooth and creamy. If the consistency is too thick, add a bit more coconut water or almond milk to thin it down.
4. Two glasses should be filled with the smoothie.

Apple Spinach Smoothie

Calories per Serving:
150

Prep Time: 5 minutes Serving Size: 2 servings

Fat: 2g

Protein: 3g

Carbs: 32g

1 green apple, cored and chopped (leave the skin on for added fiber)	1/2 cup water or coconut water for extra hydration.
1 cup fresh spinach leaves	1 tablespoon ground flaxseed
1/2 banana, peeled and sliced	1/2 lemon, juiced
1/2 cucumber, peeled and chopped	1/2 inch fresh ginger, peeled and grated
1/2 cup unsweetened almond milk	

Gluten-Free: Yes

Dairy-Free: Yes

Vegan: Yes

Nut-Free: Yes

1. Gather all the ingredients and cut the green apple, cucumber, and banana for simple mixing.
2. Add the diced green apple, fresh spinach, banana slices, cucumber, almond milk, and water to a high-speed blender. If using, add the ground flaxseed, lemon juice, and grated ginger.
3. Start the blender on low speed and gradually raise to high. Scrape down the sides of the blender as required to get a smooth smoothie. Blend until smooth. If the consistency is too thick, add a bit more water or almond milk.
4. Two glasses should be filled with the smoothie.

Beetroot Berry Smoothie

Calories per Serving: 150

Fat: 2g

Protein: 3g

Carbohydrates: 32g

Prep Time: 5 minutes Serving Size: 2 servings

1 small raw beetroot, peeled and chopped or 1/2 cup cooked beetroot, cooled.

1/2 cup orange juice (freshly squeezed if possible, for natural sweetness)

1 cup frozen mixed berries

1 tablespoon chia seeds

1/2 banana, peeled and sliced

1/2 teaspoon ground ginger

1/2 cup unsweetened almond milk

1 tablespoon lemon juice

Gluten-Free: Yes

Dairy-Free: Yes

Vegan: Yes

Nut-Free: Yes

1. Gather all the ingredients and ensure the beetroot is sliced into tiny pieces if using raw.
2. Add the diced beetroot, frozen mixed berries, banana slices, almond milk, and orange juice to a high-speed blender. If using, add the chia seeds, ground ginger, and lemon juice.
3. Start blending on low speed, then gradually raise to high. Blend until the smoothie is absolutely smooth. If required, add additional almond milk to attain your desired consistency.
4. Two glasses should be filled with the smoothie.

Cherry Almond Smoothie

Calories per Serving:
220

Prep Time: 5 minutes Serving Size: 2 servings

Fat: 9g

Protein: 5g

Carbohydrates: 32g

1 1/2 cups frozen cherries (pitted)	1/2 teaspoon ground cinnamon
1 tablespoon almond butter or sunflower seed butter for nut-free option	1 cup unsweetened almond milk
1 tablespoon ground flaxseed	1/2 cup water
1/2 banana, peeled and sliced	1/2 teaspoon vanilla extract

Gluten-Free: Yes

Dairy-Free: Yes

Vegan: Yes

Nut-Free: No

1. Gather all the ingredients, ensuring the cherries are frozen for a thick and icy smoothie
2. Add the frozen cherries, almond butter, banana slices, flaxseed, cinnamon, almond milk, and water to a high-speed blender. If using vanilla extract, add it now.
3. Start blending on low speed, gradually increasing to high. Blend until the smoothie is absolutely smooth and creamy. If the smoothie is too thick, add extra water or almond milk to attain your preferred consistency.
4. Two glasses should be filled with the smoothie.

Citrus Carrot Smoothie

Calories per Serving: 150

Fat: 2g

Protein: 2g

Carbohydrates: 32g

Prep Time: 10 minutes Serving Size: 2 servings

1 cup chopped carrots about 2 medium carrots

1 orange, peeled and segmented

1/2 cup pineapple chunks (fresh or frozen)

1/2 banana, peeled and sliced

1/2 inch fresh ginger, peeled and grated or 1/2 teaspoon ground ginger

1/2 teaspoon ground turmeric

1 cup unsweetened coconut water

1 tablespoon lemon juice (freshly squeezed)

1 teaspoon honey or maple syrup

Gluten-Free: Yes

Dairy-Free: Yes

Vegan: Yes

Nut-Free: Yes

1. Peel and cut the carrots and orange. If you're using fresh ginger and turmeric, peel and grate them.
2. Add the chopped carrots, orange segments, pineapple chunks, banana slices, grated ginger, and turmeric (if using) to a high-speed blender. Pour in the coconut water and add the lemon juice.
3. Start blending on low speed, then gradually raise to high. Blend until the mixture is smooth and creamy. If the smoothie is too thick, add additional coconut water to obtain your preferred consistency.
4. Taste the smoothie. If you want it sweeter, add honey or maple syrup and mix again.
5. Two glasses should be filled with the smoothie.

Blueberry Avocado Smoothie

Calories per Serving: 220

Fat: 12g

Protein: 4g

Carbohydrates: 28g

Prep Time: 5 minutes Serving Size: 2 servings

1 cup frozen blueberries

1/2 ripe avocado, peeled and pitted

1/2 banana, peeled and sliced

1 cup unsweetened almond milk

1 tablespoon ground flaxseed

1 teaspoon vanilla extract

1/2 teaspoon ground cinnamon

1/2 cup water

Gluten-Free: Yes

Dairy-Free: Yes

Vegan: Yes

Nut-Free: Yes

1. Gather all the ingredients, ensuring that the blueberries are frozen for a thick and creamy smoothie.
2. Add the frozen blueberries, avocado, banana slices, almond milk, and water to a high-speed blender. If using, add the ground flaxseed, vanilla essence, and cinnamon.
3. Start blending on low speed, gradually increasing to high. Blend until the smoothie is absolutely smooth and creamy. Adjust the consistency by adding additional water or almond milk if required.
4. Two glasses should be filled with the smoothie.

Green Smoothie

Calories per Serving: 170

Prep Time: 5 minutes Serving Size: 2 servings

Fat: 4g

Protein: 3g

Carbohydrates: 32g

1 cup frozen mango chunks

1 cup frozen pineapple chunks

1/2 banana, peeled and sliced

1 cup fresh spinach (or kale)

1/2 avocado, peeled and pitted

1 tablespoon ground flaxseed

1/2 teaspoon ground turmeric

1 cup coconut water

1/2 cup unsweetened coconut milk

Juice of 1/2 lime

Gluten-Free: Yes

Dairy-Free: Yes

Vegan: Yes

Nut-Free: Yes

1. Gather all ingredients and ensure the mango, pineapple, and banana are frozen for a thick, creamy smoothie.
2. Add the frozen mango chunks, pineapple chunks, banana slices, fresh spinach, avocado, flaxseed, and turmeric to a high-speed blender. Pour in the coconut water and coconut milk.
3. Start blending on low speed and gradually raise to high. Blend until the smoothie is smooth and creamy, scraping down the sides as required. If the smoothie is too thick, add extra coconut water or coconut milk to get your preferred consistency.
4. Pour the smoothie into two glasses, add a dash of lime juice if desired..

Strawberry Basil Smoothie

**Calories per Serving:
150**

Fat: 2g

Protein: 3g

Carbs: 32g

Prep Time: 5 minutes Serving Size: 2 servings

1 1/2 cups frozen strawberries

1/2 banana, peeled and sliced

1/4 cup fresh basil leaves, loosely packed

1 tablespoon chia seeds

1 teaspoon honey or maple syrup

1 cup unsweetened almond milk

1/2 cup water

1/2 teaspoon lemon juice

Gluten-Free: Yes

Dairy-Free: Yes

Vegan: Yes

Nut-Free: Yes

1. Gather all the components. Make sure the strawberries are frozen for a thick and pleasant smoothie.
2. Add the frozen strawberries, banana slices, fresh basil leaves, chia seeds, and almond milk to a high-speed blender. If using, add honey or maple syrup and lemon juice.
3. Begin with a low speed and gradually raise it to high as the blender starts to run. Blend until the smoothie is absolutely smooth and creamy. If the smoothie is too thick, add water to obtain your preferred consistency.
4. Two glasses should be filled with the smoothie.

Ginger Peach Smoothie

Calories per Serving: 170

Fat: 2g

Protein: 2g

Carbohydrates: 38g

Prep Time: 5 minutes Serving Size: 2 servings

1 1/2 cups frozen peach slices

1/2 inch fresh ginger, peeled and grated or 1/2 teaspoon ground ginger

1/2 banana, peeled and sliced

1 cup unsweetened almond milk

1 tablespoon chia seeds

1/2 teaspoon ground turmeric

1 teaspoon honey or maple syrup

Gluten-Free: Yes

Dairy-Free: Yes

Vegan: Yes

Nut-Free: Yes

1/2 cup coconut water or plain water

1. Make sure the peaches are frozen for a rich and creamy texture. Grate the fresh ginger if using, or measure the ground ginger.
2. Add the frozen peach slices, grated ginger, banana slices, almond milk, and coconut water to a high-speed blender. If used, add the chia seeds, turmeric, and honey or maple syrup.
3. Start blending on low speed, then gradually raise to high. Blend until the smoothie is absolutely smooth. Adjust the consistency by adding extra coconut water or almond milk if required.
4. Two glasses should be filled with the smoothie.

Cucumber Mint Smoothie

Calories per Serving: 90

Fat: 1g

Prep Time: 5 minutes Serving Size: 2 servings

Protein: 2g

Carbohydrates: 20g

1 cup cucumber, peeled and chopped

1/2 cup fresh mint leaves plus extra for garnish

1/2 green apple, cored and chopped

1/2 lemon, juiced

1 tablespoon chia seeds

1 cup unsweetened coconut water or plain water

1/2 teaspoon fresh ginger, peeled and grated

A few ice cubes

Gluten-Free: Yes

Dairy-Free: Yes

Vegan: Yes

Nut-Free: Yes

1. Peel and cut the cucumber and green apple. Juice the lemon. If using fresh ginger, peel and grate it.
2. Add the cucumber, mint leaves, green apple, lemon juice, chia seeds (if used), and ginger (if using) to a high-speed blender. Pour in the coconut water.
3. Start blending on low speed, then gradually raise to high. Blend until the smoothie is smooth and fully integrated. Add ice cubes if required and blend again until nicely combined.
4. Pour the smoothie into two glasses and decorate with more mint leaves if desired.

Papaya Turmeric Smoothie

**Calories per Serving:
180**

Fat: 2g

Prep Time: 5 minutes Serving Size: 2 servings

Protein: 2g

Carbs: 43g

1 1/2 cups frozen papaya chunks	**1 tablespoon chia seeds**
1/2 teaspoon ground turmeric or 1/2 inch fresh turmeric root, peeled and grated	**1/2 teaspoon ground ginger or 1/2 inch fresh ginger, peeled and grated**
1/2 ripe banana, peeled and sliced	**1/2 teaspoon honey or maple syrup**
1 cup unsweetened coconut milk	
1/2 cup orange juice	

Gluten-Free: Yes

Dairy-Free: Yes

Vegan: Yes

Nut-Free: Yes

1. Gather all the ingredients. Ensure that the papaya is frozen for a thicker, cooler smoothie.
2. Add the frozen papaya chunks, turmeric, banana slices, coconut milk, and orange juice to a high-speed blender. If using, add the chia seeds, ginger, and honey or maple syrup.
3. Start blending on low speed, then gradually raise to high. Blend until the mixture is smooth and creamy. If the smoothie is too thick, add a touch more coconut milk or orange juice to obtain your preferred consistency.
4. Two glasses should be filled with the smoothie..

Raspberry Chia Smoothie

Calories per Serving:
170

Fat: 5g

Protein: 4g

Carbs: 30g

Prep Time: 5 minutes Serving Size: 2 servings

1 cup frozen raspberries

1 tablespoon chia seeds

1/2 ripe banana, peeled and sliced

1 cup unsweetened almond milk

1/2 cup coconut water or plain water

1/2 teaspoon ground turmeric

1/2 teaspoon ground cinnamon

1 teaspoon honey or maple syrup

Gluten-Free: Yes

Dairy-Free: Yes

Vegan: Yes

Nut-Free: Yes

1. Gather all the ingredients. Ensure the raspberries are frozen to produce a thick, cool smoothie.
2. Add the frozen raspberries, chia seeds, banana slices, almond milk, and coconut water to a high-speed blender. If using, add turmeric, cinnamon, and honey or maple syrup.
3. Begin with a low speed and gradually raise it to high as the blender starts to run. Blend until the mixture is absolutely smooth. If the smoothie is too thick, add additional coconut water or almond milk to attain your preferred consistency.
4. Two glasses should be filled with the smoothie.

If you like a thicker smoothie, you may add additional chia seeds or lower the liquid.

Pomegranate Beet Smoothie

Calories per Serving: 180

Fat: 2g

Protein: 3g

Carbs: 40g

Prep Time: 10 minutes Serving Size: 2 servings

1/2 cup cooked and cooled beetroot, diced or 1/2 cup frozen beetroot chunks

1 cup pomegranate seeds or 1/2 cup pomegranate juice

1 ripe banana, peeled and sliced

1/2 cup unsweetened almond milk

1/2 cup water or more to adjust consistency

1 tablespoon chia seeds

1/2 teaspoon ground cinnamon

1/2 teaspoon ground turmeric

1/2 tablespoon fresh lemon juice

Gluten-Free: Yes

Dairy-Free: Yes

Vegan: Yes

Nut-Free: Yes

1. If using fresh beetroot, peel, cook, and chill it before dicing. If using frozen beets, ensure they are warmed sufficiently for easy mixing.
2. Add the beets, pomegranate seeds (or juice), banana, almond milk, and water to a high-speed blender. If using chia seeds, cinnamon, turmeric, and lemon juice, add them now.
3. Start blending on low speed, then gradually raise to high. Blend until the smoothie is smooth and creamy. If the smoothie is too thick, add extra water to get your preferred consistency.
4. Two glasses should be filled with the smoothie.

Kiwi Spinach Smoothie

Calories per Serving:
150

Prep Time: 5 minutes Serving Size: 2 servings

Fat: 2g

Protein: 3g

Carbs: 33g

2 ripe kiwis, peeled and sliced	1 tablespoon chia seeds
1 cup fresh spinach leaves	1/2 teaspoon ground flaxseed
1/2 banana, peeled and sliced	1/2 teaspoon lemon juice
1 cup unsweetened almond milk	
1/2 cup water or more	

Gluten-Free: Yes

Dairy-Free: Yes

Vegan: Yes

Nut-Free: Yes

1. Gather all the components. Ensure the spinach is rinsed properly, and the kiwis and banana are peeled and sliced.
2. Add the sliced kiwis, fresh spinach, banana slices, almond milk, and water to a high-speed blender. If using, add the chia seeds, ground flaxseed, and lemon juice.
3. Begin with a low speed and gradually raise it to high as the blender starts to run. Blend until the smoothie is absolutely smooth. If the smoothie is too thick, add extra water to get your preferred consistency.
4. Two glasses should be filled with the smoothie.

Orange Carrot Smoothie

Calories per Serving: 180

Prep Time: 5 minutes Serving Size: 2 servings

Fat: 3g

Protein: 2g

Carbs: 39g

1 cup fresh or frozen orange segments about 1 large orange

1/2 teaspoon ground turmeric

1 tablespoon chia seeds

1 cup fresh or frozen carrot slices about 2 medium carrots

1/4 teaspoon ground ginger

1/2 banana, peeled and sliced

1/2 teaspoon honey or maple syrup

1 cup unsweetened almond milk

Gluten-Free: Yes

1/2 cup water or more

Dairy-Free: Yes

Vegan: Yes

Nut-Free: Yes

1. Peel and slice the orange and carrots. If using fresh carrots, try boiling them moderately to maximize their blendability, but frozen carrots work well too.
2. Add the orange segments, carrot slices, banana, almond milk, and water to a high-speed blender. If using, add the turmeric, chia seeds, ground ginger, and honey or maple syrup.
3. Start blending on low speed, then gradually raise to high. Blend until the mixture is smooth and creamy. Adjust the consistency by adding additional water if required.
4. Two glasses should be filled with the smoothie.

Watermelon Mint Smoothie

Calories per Serving:
130

Prep Time: 5 minutes Serving Size: 2 servings

Fat: 0.5g

Protein: 2g

Carbs: 33g

2 cups diced seedless watermelon preferably frozen for a thicker smoothie

1 tablespoon chia seeds

1 cup unsweetened coconut water or plain water

1/4 cup fresh mint leaves, more if you like a stronger mint flavor

A few ice cubes (if using fresh watermelon instead of frozen)

1/2 cucumber, peeled and chopped

1/2 lime, juiced

Gluten-Free: Yes

Dairy-Free: Yes

Vegan: Yes

Nut-Free: Yes

1. If using fresh watermelon, you may need to add ice cubes to produce a cooled, thick thickness. Dice the watermelon and peel the cucumber.
2. Add the diced watermelon, fresh mint leaves, sliced cucumber, lime juice, chia seeds (if using), and coconut water to a high-speed blender.
3. Blend on high until the mixture is smooth and creamy. If you used fresh watermelon and need a cooler smoothie, add a few ice cubes and mix again.
4. Two glasses should be filled with the smoothie.

Apple Cinnamon Smoothie

Calories per Serving: 190

Fat: 3g

Protein: 3g

Carbohydrates: 38g

Prep Time: 5 minutes Serving Size: 2 servings

1 large apple, cored and chopped preferably organic	1 cup unsweetened almond milk
1/2 teaspoon ground cinnamon	1/2 cup water or more
1/2 banana, peeled and sliced	1/4 teaspoon ground turmeric
1 tablespoon chia seeds	1/2 teaspoon vanilla extract

Gluten-Free: Yes

Dairy-Free: Yes

Vegan: Yes

Nut-Free: Yes

1. Core and cut the apple into smaller pieces. Peel and slice the banana. Ensure that all components are ready for mixing.
2. Add the diced apple, banana slices, ground cinnamon, chia seeds (if using), almond milk, and water to a high-speed blender. If using, add the turmeric and vanilla essence.
3. Start blending on low speed and gradually raise to high. Blend until the smoothie is absolutely smooth. Adjust the consistency by adding additional water if required.
4. Two glasses should be filled with the smoothie.

CHAPTER 3

PANCAKES AND WAFFLES

Turmeric Banana Pancakes

Gingerbread Pancakes

Pumpkin Spice Pancakes

Matcha Green Tea Pancakes

Lemon Poppy Seed Pancakes

Beetroot Pancakes

Coconut Flour Waffles

Buckwheat Waffles

Flaxseed Waffles

Turmeric Waffles

Sweet Potato Waffles

Turmeric Banana Pancakes

Calories per Serving: 250

Fat: 8g

Protein: 6g

Carbohydrates: 42g

Gluten-Free: Yes

Dairy-Free: Yes

Vegan: Yes

Nut-Free: Yes

Prep Time: 10 minutes Cooking Time: 15 minutes Serving Size: 4 pancakes (2 servings)

1 ripe banana, mashed

1/2 cup gluten-free oat flour or ground oats

1/4 cup almond flour or more gluten-free oat flour for a nut-free option

1/2 teaspoon ground turmeric

1/2 teaspoon ground cinnamon

1 teaspoon baking powder (gluten-free)

1/4 teaspoon sea salt

1/2 cup unsweetened almond milk

1 tablespoon ground flaxseed mixed with 3 tablespoons water (flax egg substitute)

1 teaspoon vanilla extract

Coconut oil or avocado oil

1. To thicken, combine the ground flaxseed and water in a small dish and set aside for 5 minutes.
2. In a medium bowl, mix together the gluten-free oat flour, almond flour, turmeric, cinnamon, baking powder, and sea salt.
3. Make a smooth puree by mashing the ripe banana in a different dish. The almond milk, flax egg, and (if desired) vanilla essence should be stirred in.
4. Simply blend the dry components with the wet ones by pouring the liquids into the dry ones and stirring. A thick yet pourable batter is ideal. Add more almond milk if it's too thick.

5. Heat a non-stick pan or griddle over medium heat and gently coat with coconut oil or avocado oil. Pour 1/4 cup of the batter onto the griddle for each pancake. Cook for 2-3 minutes on each side, or until golden brown and heated through.
6. Serve the pancakes warm, topped with fresh fruit, a drizzle of maple syrup, or a sprinkling of more cinnamon.

These pancakes may be kept in the refrigerator for up to 3 days and reheated for a quick breakfast.

Gingerbread Pancakes

Calories per Serving: 200

Fat: 7g

Protein: 4g

Carbohydrates: 32g

Prep Time: 10 minutes Cooking Time: 15 minutes Serving Size: 4 servings (makes about 8 pancakes)

Gluten-Free: Yes

Dairy-Free: Yes

Vegan: Yes

Nut-Free: Yes

1 cup gluten-free all-purpose flour or regular if not gluten-free

1 teaspoon baking powder

1/2 teaspoon baking soda

1 teaspoon ground ginger

1 teaspoon ground cinnamon

1/4 teaspoon ground cloves

1/4 teaspoon ground nutmeg

1/4 teaspoon salt

2 tablespoons ground flaxseed mixed with 6 tablespoons water or 2 large eggs for non-vegan

1/4 cup unsweetened applesauce

1/4 cup molasses

1 cup unsweetened almond milk

2 tablespoons coconut oil, melted plus extra for cooking

1 teaspoon vanilla extract

1. In a small dish, blend the ground flaxseed with water and let it rest for approximately 5 minutes until it thickens. If you're not preparing vegan pancakes, you may skip this step and use 2 eggs instead.
2. In a large mixing bowl, whisk together the gluten-free flour, baking powder, baking soda, ground ginger, cinnamon, cloves, nutmeg, and salt.

3. In another dish, mix together the flaxseed egg (or normal eggs), applesauce, molasses, almond milk, melted coconut oil, and vanilla extract.
4. Pour the wet ingredients into the dry ingredients and gently whisk until just incorporated. The batter should be thick, but if it's too thick, add a bit more almond milk to obtain the appropriate consistency.
5. Heat a large non-stick pan or griddle over medium heat and gently coat with coconut oil. Pour roughly 1/4 cup of batter each pancake onto the skillet. Cook until bubbles form on the top, approximately 2-3 minutes, then turn and cook for another 2-3 minutes until golden brown and cooked through.
6. Serve warm with your favorite toppings, such as maple syrup, fresh fruit, or a dollop of coconut yogurt.

Make sure to use gluten-free flour if you require the pancakes to be gluten-free. There are several good gluten-free all-purpose flour mixes available.

.

Pumpkin Spice Pancakes

**Calories per Serving:
180**

Fat: 6g

Protein: 4g

Carbohydrates: 28g

Gluten-Free: Yes

Dairy-Free: Yes

Vegan: Yes

Nut-Free: Yes

Prep Time: 10 minutes Cooking Time: 15 minutes Serving Size: 4 servings (makes about 8 pancakes)

1 cup gluten-free oat flour or a mix of almond flour and gluten-free all-purpose flour

1/2 cup canned pumpkin puree, make sure it's pure pumpkin, not pie filling

1 tablespoon ground flaxseed + 3 tablespoons water (for a flax egg)

1 tablespoon maple syrup

1 teaspoon baking powder

1/2 teaspoon baking soda

1 teaspoon ground cinnamon

1/2 teaspoon ground ginger

1/4 teaspoon ground nutmeg

1/4 teaspoon ground cloves

1/2 teaspoon ground turmeric

1/4 teaspoon salt

1/2 teaspoon vanilla extract

3/4 cup unsweetened almond milk

1 tablespoon coconut oil plus extra for the pan

1. In a small dish, blend the ground flaxseed with 3 tablespoons of water. Stir and let it rest for approximately 5 minutes to thicken.
2. In a large mixing basin, whisk together the oat flour, baking powder, baking soda, and cinnamon, ginger, nutmeg, cloves, turmeric, and salt.
3. In another dish, mix together the pumpkin puree, flax egg, maple syrup, vanilla extract, and almond milk until smooth.
4. Simply blend the dry components with the wet ones by pouring the liquids into the dry ones and stirring. A thick yet

pourable batter is ideal. Add more almond milk if it's too thick.

5. Heat a non-stick pan or griddle over medium heat and gently coat with coconut oil. Pour 1/4 cup of batter into the griddle for each pancake. Cook for 2-3 minutes until bubbles develop on the surface and the edges appear set. Flip and cook for another 2-3 minutes on the other side until golden brown and cooked through. Adjust heat as required to avoid burning.

6. Serve the pancakes warm, topped with a drizzle of maple syrup, a sprinkling of cinnamon, or your favorite toppings.

Matcha Green Tea Pancakes

Calories per Serving: 160

Fat: 7g

Protein: 4g

Carbohydrates: 22g

Prep Time: 10 minutes Cooking Time: 15 minutes Serving Size: 4 servings (8 small pancakes)

1 cup gluten-free all-purpose flour or almond flour for a lower-carb option

1 tablespoon matcha green tea powder (culinary grade)

1 tablespoon ground flaxseed

1 tablespoon coconut sugar or maple syrup

1 teaspoon baking powder

1/4 teaspoon baking soda

1/4 teaspoon sea salt

1 cup unsweetened almond milk

1 tablespoon apple cider vinegar

1 teaspoon vanilla extract

2 tablespoons coconut oil, melted

Gluten-Free: Yes

Dairy-Free: Yes

Vegan: Optional

1. In a large mixing bowl, whisk together the gluten-free flour, matcha powder, powdered flaxseed, coconut sugar, baking powder, baking soda, and sea salt
2. In a separate dish, combine the almond milk and apple cider vinegar. Let it rest for a minute to curdle slightly (this forms a vegan "buttermilk"). Then, add the vanilla extract and melted coconut oil to the almond milk mixture.
3. Pour the wet components into the dry ingredients, stirring gently until just incorporated. Be cautious not to overmix; the batter should be somewhat lumpy.
4. Heat a non-stick pan or griddle over medium heat and gently coat with coconut oil. Pour approximately 1/4 cup of batter into the griddle for each pancake. Cook until bubbles form on

the top, then turn and cook the other side until golden brown, approximately 2-3 minutes each side.

5. Serve the pancakes warm, topped with your choice of fresh berries, a drizzle of maple syrup, or a dollop of coconut yogurt for additional richness.

Lemon Poppy Seed Pancakes

Calories per Serving: 180

Fat: 7g

Protein: 4g

Carbohydrates: 25g

Prep Time: 10 minutes Cooking Time: 15 minutes Serving Size: 4 servings (makes about 8 pancakes)

1 cup gluten-free flour blend ensure it includes xanthan gum or similar binding agent

1 tablespoon poppy seeds

2 tablespoons coconut sugar or another natural sweetener

1 teaspoon baking powder

1/2 teaspoon baking soda

1/4 teaspoon sea salt

1 tablespoon lemon zest (from 1-2 lemons)

1 tablespoon fresh lemon juice

3/4 cup unsweetened almond milk

1 tablespoon apple cider vinegar

2 tablespoons melted coconut oil or olive oil

1 teaspoon vanilla extract

Optional Additions:

1 tablespoon ground flaxseed

Fresh berries

Gluten-Free: Yes

**Dairy-Free: Yes

Vegan: Yes

Nut-Free: Yes

1. In a small dish, mix the almond milk and apple cider vinegar, and let it rest for a few minutes to produce a vegan "buttermilk." Then, whisk in the lemon juice, lemon zest, melted coconut oil, and vanilla essence.
2. In a large mixing bowl, whisk together the gluten-free flour, poppy seeds, coconut sugar, baking powder, baking soda, and sea salt. If using, add the ground flaxseed.
3. Pour the wet ingredients into the dry ingredients and gently stir until just mixed. Be cautious not to overmix the batter; it's good if a few lumps remain.
4. Heat a non-stick skillet or griddle over medium heat. Lightly coat it with coconut oil or olive oil. Pour approximately 1/4 cup of batter into the griddle for each pancake. Cook for 2-3 minutes on each side, or until bubbles appear on the top and the edges are firm, then turn and cook for another 2 minutes until golden brown.
5. Serve the pancakes warm, topped with fresh berries, a drizzle of maple syrup, or a dollop of dairy-free yogurt.

Beetroot Pancakes

Calories per Serving: 150

Prep Time: 15 minutes Cooking Time: 20 minutes Serving Size: 4 servings (8 pancakes)

Fat: 5g

Protein: 4g

Carbohydrates: 24g

1 medium beetroot, peeled and grated about 1/2 cup

1 cup gluten-free oat flour or gluten-free all-purpose flour

1 teaspoon baking powder

1/2 teaspoon ground cinnamon

1/4 teaspoon ground ginger

1/4 teaspoon salt

1 tablespoon ground flaxseed mixed with 3 tablespoons water (flax egg, or use 1 egg)

1 tablespoon maple syrup or any natural sweetener

1/2 cup unsweetened almond milk

1 tablespoon coconut oil, melted

1 teaspoon vanilla extract

Gluten-Free: Yes

Dairy-Free: Yes

Vegan: Yes

Nut-Free: Yes

1. Mix the ground flaxseed with water and put aside to thicken (if using a flax egg).
2. In a large mixing basin, combine the gluten-free oat flour, baking powder, powdered cinnamon, ground ginger (if using), and salt.
3. In another dish, mix together the flax egg (or normal egg), maple syrup, almond milk, melted coconut oil, and vanilla extract.
4. Simply blend the dry components with the wet ones by pouring the liquids into the dry ones and stirring. Fold in the grated beetroot until well distributed.
5. Heat a non-stick pan or griddle over medium heat and gently coat with coconut oil. Pour approximately 1/4 cup of batter into the griddle for each pancake. Cook for 2-3 minutes on

each side or until bubbles appear on the surface and the edges are firm.

6. Serve the pancakes warm, topped with fresh fruit, a dollop of coconut yogurt, or a drizzle of maple syrup.

If you like a smoother texture, you may purée the shredded beetroot before adding it to the batter.

To make this dish nut-free, use a nut-free milk replacement like oat milk and omit the almond milk.

Coconut Flour Waffles

Calories per Waffle:
150

Fat: 10g

Protein: 5g

Carbohydrates: 10g

Prep Time: 10 minutes Cooking Time: 10 minutes Serving Size: 4
waffles

1/2 cup coconut flour

4 large eggs (for vegan: substitute
with 4 flax eggs, see note below)

1/2 cup unsweetened almond milk

1/4 cup melted coconut oil

1 tablespoon honey or maple syrup

1 teaspoon vanilla extract

1/2 teaspoon baking soda

1/4 teaspoon sea salt

1/2 teaspoon ground
cinnamon

Gluten-Free: Yes

Dairy-Free: Yes

Vegan: No

Nut-Free: Yes

1. Gather all the ingredients and preheat your waffle iron.
2. In a large mixing bowl, whisk together the eggs (or flax eggs),
   almond milk, melted coconut oil, honey or maple syrup, and
   vanilla extract until smooth.
3. Add the coconut flour, baking soda, sea salt, and cinnamon to
   the wet ingredients. Stir until completely blended. The dough
   will be thick owing to the coconut flour's absorbent nature.
4. Lightly lubricate the waffle iron with a little coconut oil to
   avoid sticking. Pour the batter into the prepared waffle iron,
   spreading it out evenly. Cook for approximately 3-5 minutes,
   or until the waffles are golden brown and crispy on the edges.
5. Remove the waffles from the iron and serve immediately with
   your favorite toppings like fresh berries, a dollop of coconut
   yogurt, or a drizzle of honey.

Flax Eggs: To create a flax egg, combine 1 tablespoon of ground flaxseed with 3 tablespoons of water. Let it rest for 5 minutes to thicken. This recipe takes 4 flax eggs for creating vegan waffles.

Coconut Flour is quite absorbent, therefore it's crucial to measure it correctly. The batter will be thicker than regular waffle batter.

Honey or Maple Syrup may be eliminated for a lower-sugar alternative.

Buckwheat Waffles

Calories per Serving: 220

Fat: 8g

Protein: 6g

Carbohydrates: 33g

Prep Time: 10 minutes Cooking Time: 15 minutes Serving Size: 4 waffles

1 cup buckwheat flour

1 tablespoon ground flaxseed + 3 tablespoons water (flax egg)

1 tablespoon coconut oil, melted plus more for greasing the waffle iron

1 cup unsweetened almond milk

1 tablespoon maple syrup or honey for non-vegan

1 teaspoon baking powder

1/2 teaspoon ground cinnamon

1/4 teaspoon sea salt

1/2 teaspoon vanilla extract

Gluten-Free: Yes

Dairy-Free: Yes

Vegan: Yes

1. In a small dish, combine the ground flaxseed with water. Let it rest for approximately 5 minutes to thicken.
2. In a large basin, mix together the buckwheat flour, baking powder, cinnamon, and sea salt.
3. In a separate dish, combine the almond milk, melted coconut oil, maple syrup, vanilla extract, and the prepared flax egg.
4. Simply blend the dry components with the wet ones by pouring the liquids into the dry ones and stirring. Be cautious not to overmix; a few lumps are alright.
5. Preheat your waffle iron according to the manufacturer's directions. Lightly grease it with coconut oil.
6. Pour the batter into the hot waffle iron, spreading it evenly. Close the waffle iron and cook for approximately 5 minutes, or until the waffles are golden brown and cooked through.

7. Carefully take the waffles from the iron and serve warm with your favorite toppings like fresh berries, a sprinkle of maple syrup, or almond butter.

These waffles freeze nicely, so try preparing a double batch and saving leftovers for quick breakfasts.

Flaxseed Waffles

Calories per Serving: 230

Fat: 14g

Protein: 6g

Carbohydrates: 20g

Prep Time: 10 minutes Cooking Time: 15 minutes Serving Size: 4 servings (makes about 4 waffles)

1 cup gluten-free oat flour or almond flour for a lower-carb option

1/4 cup ground flaxseeds

1 teaspoon baking powder

1/2 teaspoon ground cinnamon

1/4 teaspoon salt

1 cup unsweetened almond milk

2 tablespoons coconut oil, melted or avocado oil

1 tablespoon maple syrup

1 teaspoon vanilla extract

2 tablespoons apple cider vinegar or lemon juice

1 flax egg (1 tablespoon ground flaxseed mixed with 3 tablespoons water, let sit for 5 minutes) or 1 large egg (if not vegan)

Gluten-Free: Yes

Dairy-Free: Yes

Vegan: Yes

Nut-Free: Yes

1. In a small dish, combine 1 tablespoon ground flaxseed with 3 tablespoons of water. Stir and let rest for approximately 5 minutes until it thickens.
2. In a large basin, mix together the oat flour, ground flaxseeds, baking powder, cinnamon, and salt.
3. In another dish, add the almond milk, melted coconut oil, maple syrup, vanilla extract, and apple cider vinegar. Add the flax egg or normal egg and stir until fully blended.
4. Simply blend the dry components with the wet ones by pouring the liquids into the dry ones and stirring. Be cautious not to overmix; the batter should be somewhat thick.
5. Preheat your waffle iron according to the manufacturer's directions.

6. Lightly grease the waffle iron with a touch of coconut oil or non-stick spray. Pour the batter into the waffle iron, spreading it out evenly. Cook according to your waffle iron's directions, generally around 3-5 minutes, until the waffles are golden brown and crisp.

7. Serve the waffles warm with your favorite toppings such as fresh berries, sliced bananas, a drizzle of maple syrup, or a sprinkling of extra ground flaxseeds.

Using Oat Flour makes the waffles gluten-free while offering a wonderful amount of fiber.

Apple Cider Vinegar Or lemon juice combines with the baking powder to make the waffles rise and become fluffy.

Turmeric Waffles

Calories per Serving: 220

Fat: 10g

Protein: 5g

Carbohydrates: 28g

Prep Time: 10 minutes Cooking Time: 15 minutes Serving Size: 4 waffles

1 cup gluten-free oat flour or any gluten-free flour blend

1 tablespoon ground turmeric

1 teaspoon ground cinnamon

1 tablespoon ground flaxseed or chia seeds

2 tablespoons coconut sugar

1 teaspoon baking powder

1/4 teaspoon baking soda

1/4 teaspoon sa1 cup unsweetened almond milk

1 tablespoon apple cider vinegar

2 tablespoons coconut oil, melted

1 teaspoon vanilla extract

1 large egg (or flax egg for vegan: 1 tablespoon ground flaxseed + 3 tablespoons water, mixed and left to sit for 5 minutes)

Gluten-Free: Yes

Dairy-Free: Yes

Vegan: Yes

Nut-Free: Yes

1. Preheat your waffle iron according to the manufacturer's directions.
2. In a large bowl, mix together the oat flour, ground turmeric, cinnamon, powdered flaxseed, coconut sugar, baking powder, baking soda, and salt.
3. In a separate dish, combine the almond milk and apple cider vinegar. Let it rest for a minute to curdle slightly (this functions like buttermilk). Then, add the melted coconut oil, vanilla essence, and the egg (or flax egg if vegan). Whisk until thoroughly blended.
4. Pour the wet components into the dry ingredients. Stir until just blended, being careful not to overmix. A thick yet

pourable batter is ideal. If it's too thick, add a touch more almond milk.

5. Lightly grease the waffle iron with a touch of coconut oil or non-stick spray. Pour the mixture into the waffle iron and cook according to your waffle iron's directions, normally approximately 3-5 minutes per waffle, until golden and crisp

6. Serve the waffles warm with your favorite anti-inflammatory toppings like fresh berries, a drizzle of honey or maple syrup, and a sprinkle of additional cinnamon or turmeric.

For a Crispier Waffle, Cook a bit longer till golden brown.

Sweet Potato Waffles

Calories per Waffle: 120

Fat: 4g

Protein: 2g

Carbohydrates: 20g

Prep Time: 15 minutes Cooking Time: 15 minutes Serving Size: 4 waffles

1 medium sweet potato, peeled and cubed about 1 cup

1 tablespoon ground flaxseed mixed with 3 tablespoons water to form a flax egg

1/2 cup almond flour

1/4 cup coconut flour

1/2 teaspoon ground cinnamon

1/4 teaspoon ground turmeric

1/4 teaspoon baking powder

1/4 teaspoon sea salt

1/2 teaspoon vanilla extract

1/2 cup unsweetened almond milk

Gluten-Free: Yes

Dairy-Free: Yes

Vegan: Yes

Remove the steaks from the refrigerator and let them sit for about half an hour to come to room temperature. This guarantees uniform cooking..

Lightly season the steaks on both sides with salt and pepper.r.

Turn up the heat to high and thoroughly heat the cast iron skillet. Prior to adding the meat, the pan should be slightly smoking.

CHAPTER 4

EGGS AND POTATOES

Spinach and Sweet Potato Frittata

Scrambled Eggs with Sweet Potatoes

Sweet Potato Hash with Eggs

Egg and Sweet Potato Tacos

Baked Eggs in Potato Nests

Sweet Potato and Spinach Skillet

Egg and Sweet Potato Burrito

Sweet Potato and Egg Casserole

Roasted Potatoes with Poached Eggs

Egg and Sweet Potato Muffins

Spinach and Sweet Potato Frittata

Calories per Serving: 220

Fat: 11g

Protein: 10g

Carbohydrates: 20g

Gluten-Free: Yes

Dairy-Free: Yes

Vegetarian: Yes

Nut-Free: Yes

Prep Time: 10 minutes Cooking Time: 30 minutes Serving Size: 4 servings

1 medium sweet potato, peeled and thinly sliced

2 cups fresh spinach leaves

1 small onion, finely chopped

6 large eggs

1/4 cup unsweetened almond milk

1 tablespoon olive oil or avocado oil

1/2 teaspoon turmeric powder

1/4 teaspoon ground black pepper

1/4 teaspoon sea salt or to taste

1/4 teaspoon smoked paprika

Fresh herbs like parsley or chives

1. Preheat your oven to 375°F (190°C).
2. Heat olive oil in a large oven-safe skillet over medium heat. Add the thinly sliced sweet potato and cook for approximately 5-7 minutes until they start to soften, turning periodically.
3. Add the chopped onions to the pan and sauté for another 3-4 minutes until transparent. Then, add the spinach and simmer until wilted, approximately 2 minutes.
4. In a medium bowl, mix together the eggs, almond milk, turmeric, black pepper, and salt until thoroughly incorporated.
5. Pour the egg mixture over the sautéed veggies in the pan, ensuring the eggs are equally distributed. If using smoked paprika, sprinkle it over top.
6. Allow the frittata to cook on the stovetop for 2-3 minutes until the edges start to firm. Then, move the pan to the preheated

oven and bake for 15-20 minutes, or until the eggs are all set and the top is brown.

7. Remove from the oven and let it cool somewhat before slicing. Garnish with fresh herbs if desired.

To make the recipe dairy-free, use plant-based milk and omit the cheese. You may also add nutritional yeast for a cheese taste.

Scrambled Eggs with Sweet Potatoes

Calories per Serving: 300

Fat: 16g

Protein: 12g

Carbohydrates: 28g

Prep Time: 10 minutes Cooking Time: 20 minutes Serving Size: 2 servings

2 medium sweet potatoes, peeled and diced

4 large eggs

1/2 teaspoon ground turmeric

1/4 teaspoon ground black pepper

1/4 teaspoon ground cumin

1 tablespoon olive oil or coconut oil

1/4 cup onion, finely chopped

1 garlic clove, minced

1/2 cup baby spinach

Salt to taste

Fresh parsley or cilantro

Gluten-Free: Yes

Dairy-Free: Yes

Nut-Free: Yes

Prepare Sweet Potatoes:

1. Preheat the oven to 400°F (200°C).
2. Toss the chopped sweet potatoes with 1/2 tablespoon of olive oil and a sprinkle of salt. Spread them out on a baking sheet.
3. Roast for approximately 20 minutes, rotating halfway through, until the sweet potatoes are soft and slightly caramelized.

Cook the Scrambled Eggs:

4. While the sweet potatoes are roasting, heat the remaining 1/2 tablespoon of olive oil in a non-stick pan over medium heat.
5. Add the chopped onion and sauté until it turns translucent, approximately 3-4 minutes.
6. Add the minced garlic and simmer for another minute.

7. In a small bowl, mix together the eggs, turmeric, black pepper, cumin, and a touch of salt.

8. Pour the egg mixture into the skillet with the onions and garlic. Stir continually until the eggs are lightly scrambled.

9. If using, add the baby spinach during the final minute of cooking, stirring until wilted.

Assemble and Serve:

10. Divide the cooked sweet potatoes between two dishes.

11. Top each platter with the turmeric scrambled eggs.

12. Garnish with fresh parsley or cilantro, if preferred.

Sweet Potato Hash with Eggs

Calories per Serving: 250

Fat: 12g

Protein: 10g

Carbohydrates: 28g

Prep Time: 10 minutes Cooking Time: 20 minutes Serving Size: 4 servings

2 medium sweet potatoes, peeled and diced into small cubes

1 red bell pepper, diced

1 small red onion, diced

2 tablespoons olive oil

1/2 teaspoon ground turmeric

1/2 teaspoon ground cumin

1/2 teaspoon smoked paprika

Salt and black pepper to taste

4 large eggs or use tofu/chickpeas for a vegan option

2 tablespoons chopped fresh parsley

Gluten-Free: Yes

Dairy-Free: Yes

Vegan: No

1. Dice the sweet potatoes, red bell pepper, and red onion into tiny, consistent pieces to promote even cooking.
2. Heat 2 tablespoons of olive oil in a large pan over medium heat. Add the diced sweet potatoes and simmer for approximately 10 minutes, stirring periodically, until they start to soften.
3. Add the diced red bell pepper and red onion to the pan with the sweet potatoes. Stir in the turmeric, cumin, smoked paprika, salt, and pepper. Continue to boil for another 5-7 minutes, or until the sweet potatoes are soft and the veggies are cooked through.
4. Make 4 tiny wells in the sweet potato hash mixture in the pan. Crack one egg into each well (or add tofu/chickpeas if creating a vegan variation). Cover the pan with a cover and heat for 3-4 minutes, or until the egg whites are set but the yolks are still runny. Cook longer if you desire completely set yolks.

5. Once the eggs are cooked to your taste, remove the pan from heat. Garnish with chopped fresh parsley, if using. Serve immediately.

For a Vegan Option, skip the eggs and substitute them with tofu or chickpeas for a plant-based protein source.

Egg and Sweet Potato Tacos

Calories per Serving: 300

Fat: 15g

Protein: 10g

Carbohydrates: 32g

Prep Time: 10 minutes Cooking Time: 20 minutes Serving Size: 4 tacos (2 servings)

Gluten-Free: Yes

Dairy-Free: Yes

Vegetarian: Yes

1 medium sweet potato, peeled and diced

1 tablespoon olive oil

1/2 teaspoon ground cumin

1/2 teaspoon paprika

1/2 teaspoon turmeric

Salt and pepper

4 large eggs

4 small corn tortillas

1/2 avocado, sliced

1/4 cup fresh cilantro, chopped

1 tablespoon lime juice

Dairy-free cheese, salsa, or hot sauce

Prepare Sweet Potatoes:

1. Preheat the oven to 400°F (200°C).
2. Toss the chopped sweet potatoes with olive oil, cumin, paprika, turmeric, salt, and pepper.
3. Spread them out on a baking sheet and roast for 20 minutes, or until soft and slightly crispy on the edges.

Cook Eggs:

4. While the sweet potatoes are roasting, break the eggs into a basin, season with salt and pepper, and whisk thoroughly.

5. Heat a non-stick pan over medium heat and cook the eggs, scrambling them until thoroughly done.

6. Warm Tortillas: Heat the tortillas on a dry pan or microwave them for approximately 20 seconds to soften.

Assemble Tacos:

7. Lay out the heated tortillas and distribute the roasted sweet potatoes and scrambled eggs among them.
8. Top with avocado slices, fresh cilantro, and a sprinkle of lime juice.
9. Add extra toppings like dairy-free cheese, salsa, or spicy sauce if preferred.
10. Serve the tacos warm

To make this dish dairy-free, eliminate the cheese or use a plant-based replacement. For a hotter kick, add extra hot sauce or salsa.

Baked Eggs in Potato Nests

Calories per Serving: 180

Fat: 10g

Protein: 8g

Carbohydrates: 15g

Prep Time: 10 minutes Cooking Time: 20 minutes Serving Size: 4 servings (2 nests per serving)

2 medium sweet potatoes, peeled and grated

4 large eggs

2 tablespoons olive oil

1/2 teaspoon ground turmeric

1/2 teaspoon ground cumin

1/2 teaspoon paprika

1/4 teaspoon black pepper

1/2 teaspoon sea salt

Fresh herbs

Gluten-Free: Yes

Dairy-Free: Yes

Nut-Free: Yes

1. Preheat your oven to 375°F (190°C). Grease a regular muffin tray with olive oil or non-stick spray.
2. In a large bowl, mix the grated sweet potatoes with olive oil, turmeric, cumin, paprika, black pepper, and sea salt. Mix well to properly coat the sweet potatoes with the seasonings.
3. Divide the sweet potato mixture equally among the muffin pan cups, pushing the mixture down firmly and producing a nest shape with a well in the middle for the eggs.
4. Place the muffin tray in the preheated oven and bake for approximately 10 minutes, or until the sweet potato nests start to crisp up a little.
5. Remove the muffin pan from the oven. Carefully break one egg into each sweet potato nest.
6. Return the muffin tray to the oven and bake for another 10 minutes or until the egg whites are set, and the yolks are cooked to your preferred doneness.

7. Carefully remove the baked eggs in sweet potato nests from the muffin tray using a spoon or spatula. Garnish with fresh herbs if preferred, and serve warm.

Adjust the cooking time depending on your choice for egg yolk doneness—less time for runnier yolks, and longer time for completely cooked yolks.

Sweet Potato and Spinach Skillet

Calories per Serving: 280

Fat: 12g

Protein: 10g

Carbohydrates: 36g

Prep Time: 10 minutes Cooking Time: 20 minutes Serving Size: 2 servings

1 medium sweet potato, peeled and diced (2 cups)

1 tablespoon olive oil or avocado oil

1/2 small red onion, diced

1 clove garlic, minced

2 cups fresh spinach leaves

1/2 teaspoon ground turmeric

1/2 teaspoon smoked paprika

Salt and pepper to taste

2 large eggs

1 avocado, sliced

Gluten-Free: Yes

Dairy-Free: Yes

Vegan: No

Nut-Free: Yes

1. Preheat your oven to 375°F (190°C). Grease a regular muffin tray with olive oil or non-stick spray.
2. In a large bowl, mix the grated sweet potatoes with olive oil, turmeric, cumin, paprika, black pepper, and sea salt. Mix well to properly coat the sweet potatoes with the seasonings.
3. Divide the sweet potato mixture equally among the muffin pan cups, pushing the mixture down firmly and producing a nest shape with a well in the middle for the eggs.
4. Place the muffin tray in the preheated oven and bake for approximately 10 minutes, or until the sweet potato nests start to crisp up a little.
5. Remove the muffin pan from the oven. Carefully break one egg into each sweet potato nest.
6. Return the muffin tray to the oven and bake for another 10 minutes or until the egg whites are set, and the yolks are cooked to your preferred doneness.

7. Carefully remove the baked eggs in sweet potato nests from the muffin tray using a spoon or spatula. Garnish with fresh herbs if preferred, and serve warm.

Adjust the cooking time depending on your choice for egg yolk doneness—less time for runnier yolks, and longer time for completely cooked yolks.

Egg and Sweet Potato Burrito

Calories per Serving: 350

Fat: 16g

Protein: 14g

Carbohydrates: 38g

Gluten-Free: Optional

Dairy-Free: Yes

Vegetarian: Yes

Nut-Free: Yes

Prep Time: 10 minutes Cooking Time: 20 minutes Serving Size: 2 servings

1 medium sweet potato, peeled and diced

4 large eggs

1 tablespoon olive oil

1/2 teaspoon ground turmeric

1/2 teaspoon ground cumin

1/2 teaspoon smoked paprika

1/4 teaspoon black pepper

1/4 teaspoon sea salt

2 gluten-free tortillas or regular flour tortillas if not gluten-free

1/2 avocado, sliced

1/4 cup chopped fresh cilantro

Salsa

Cook Sweet Potatoes:

1. Heat olive oil in a medium pan over medium heat.
2. Add the diced sweet potatoes and simmer for approximately 10-12 minutes, turning periodically, until they are soft and slightly crispy on the outside.
3. Season with turmeric, cumin, smoked paprika, black pepper, and sea salt. Stir to coat the sweet potatoes evenly with the spices. Remove from the pan and put aside.

4. Scramble the Eggs: In the same skillet, break the eggs and scramble them over medium-low heat until thoroughly done.

You may season the eggs with a touch of salt and pepper if preferred. Remove from heat.

Assemble the Burritos:

5. **Warm the gluten-free tortillas in a dry pan or microwave until malleable.**
6. **Divide the sweet potatoes and scrambled eggs between the two tortillas.**
7. **Add avocado slices on top of the eggs and sweet potatoes for added creaminess and healthy fats.**
8. **Sprinkle with chopped fresh cilantro, if using.**

9. **Roll the Burritos: Fold the edges of the tortilla over the filling, then roll it up from the bottom to surround the contents fully. - If desired, briefly toast the burritos in the pan until golden brown on both sides for added crispiness.**

10. **Serve: Cut each tortilla in half and serve immediately with your favorite salsa on the side.**

Gluten-Free Tortillas may be used to keep the meal gluten-free

Sweet Potato and Egg Casserole

Calories per Serving: 220

Fat: 10g

Protein: 10g

Carbohydrates: 25g

Prep Time: 15 minutes Cooking Time: 45 minutes Serving Size: 6 servings

2 medium sweet potatoes, peeled and diced into small cubes

1 tablespoon olive oil

1 small onion, finely chopped

1 red bell pepper, diced

1 yellow bell pepper, diced

Gluten-Free: Yes

1 teaspoon ground turmeric

Dairy-Free: Yes

1 teaspoon smoked paprika

Vegetarian: Yes

Nut-Free: Yes

1/2 teaspoon ground cumin

Salt and pepper

6 large eggs

1/4 cup unsweetened almond milk

2 cups fresh spinach, chopped

1/4 cup chopped green onions

1. **Preheat your oven to 375°F (190°C). Grease a 9x13-inch baking dish with olive oil or non-stick spray.**
2. **In a large skillet, heat the olive oil over medium heat. Add the diced sweet potatoes and simmer for approximately 10 minutes, stirring periodically, until they start to soften.**
3. **Add the diced onion, red bell pepper, and yellow bell pepper to the pan with the sweet potatoes. Cook for another 5-7 minutes, until the veggies are softened.**
4. **Stir in the ground turmeric, smoked paprika, cumin, salt, and pepper. Mix well to coat the veggies with the seasonings. Remove from heat and put aside.**
5. **In a large dish, mix together the eggs and almond milk. Season with a little salt and pepper. Add the chopped spinach to the egg mixture and swirl to incorporate**

6. Transfer the cooked veggies to the prepared baking dish, spreading them out evenly. Pour the egg mixture over the top, ensuring the spinach is equally distributed.
7. Place the casserole in the preheated oven and bake for 30-35 minutes, or until the eggs are completely set and the top is brown.
8. Remove from the oven and let it cool somewhat before slicing. Garnish with chopped green onions if desired. Serve warm.

For additional Protein, you may put in cooked turkey sausage or crushed tofu before baking.

Roasted Potatoes with Poached Eggs

Calories per Serving: 280

Fat: 12g

Protein: 11g

Carbohydrates: 32g

Prep Time: 10 minutes Cooking Time: 30 minutes Serving Size: 2 servings

Gluten-Free: Yes

Dairy-Free: Yes

Vegetarian: Yes

Nut-Free: Yes

For the Turmeric Roasted Potatoes:

2 medium potatoes, cut into 1-inch cubes (Yukon Gold or red potatoes work well)

1 tablespoon olive oil

1/2 teaspoon ground turmeric

1/2 teaspoon ground cumin

1/2 teaspoon garlic powder

1/4 teaspoon smoked paprika

Salt and black pepper

For the Poached Eggs:

4 large eggs

1 tablespoon white vinegar

Garnishes:

Fresh parsley or cilantro, chopped

A sprinkle of red pepper flakes

Avocado slices

1. Preheat the oven to 400°F (200°C).
2. In a large mixing basin, toss the potato cubes with olive oil, turmeric, cumin, garlic powder, smoked paprika, salt, and black pepper until equally coated.
3. Spread the seasoned potatoes in a single layer on a baking sheet coated with parchment paper. Roast in the preheated oven for 25-30 minutes, rotating halfway through, until the potatoes are golden brown and crispy.
4. While the potatoes are roasting, put a medium pot of water to a slow simmer over medium heat. Add the vinegar (if using).

5. Crack one egg into a small bowl, then carefully slip it into the heating water. Repeat with the remaining eggs. Poach the eggs for 3-4 minutes, or until the whites are set but the yolks are still runny. Use a slotted spoon to delicately remove the eggs and drain on a paper towel.
6. Divide the roasted potatoes between two plates. Top each platter with two poached eggs. Garnish with fresh parsley or cilantro, red pepper flakes, and avocado slices if preferred.

Poaching eggs may be tough; adding vinegar to the water helps the eggs keep their form.

Egg and Sweet Potato Muffins

Equipment Needed:

Cast iron skillet or heavy-bottomed frying pan

Tongs

Spatula

Meat thermometer (optional)

Prep Time: 15 minutes Cooking Time: 25 minutes Serving Size: 12 muffins

1 medium sweet potato, peeled and grated (about 1 cup)

8 large eggs

1/2 cup chopped spinach

1/4 cup chopped red bell pepper

1/4 cup chopped onion

1/2 teaspoon turmeric

1/2 teaspoon ground cumin

1/4 teaspoon ground black pepper

1/4 teaspoon sea salt

1 tablespoon olive oil or coconut oil, for greasing the muffin tin

Fresh herbs

(per serving):

Calories: 520

Fat: 41.5g

Protein: 37g

Carbs: 1g

1. Preheat your oven to 350°F (175°C). Lightly butter a 12-cup muffin tray with olive oil or coconut oil.
2. Peel and shred the sweet potato. Set aside.
3. In a medium skillet, heat a tiny quantity of oil over medium heat. Add the chopped onion, red bell pepper, and shredded sweet potato. Sauté for approximately 5 minutes until the veggies are slightly softened. Add the chopped spinach and simmer for another 1-2 minutes until wilted. Remove from heat.
4. In a large mixing basin, whisk the eggs. Add the turmeric, cumin, black pepper, and sea salt. Mix until completely blended.
5. Add the sautéed veggies to the egg mixture and whisk to incorporate.

6. Pour the egg and vegetable mixture equally into the prepared muffin tray, filling each cup approximately three-quarters full.
7. Place the muffin tray in the preheated oven and bake for 20-25 minutes, or until the muffins are firm and gently brown on top.
8. Allow the muffins to cool in the tray for a few minutes before removing them. Garnish with fresh herbs if preferred, and serve warm.

These muffins may be prepared in advance and kept in the refrigerator for up to 5 days, making them excellent for meal prep.

CHAPTER 5

SALADS, WRAPS AND SANDWICHES

Berry Spinach Salad

Turmeric Chickpea Salad

Beet and Arugula Salad

Apple Walnut Salad

Chicken and Spinach Wrap

Falafel Wrap

Black Bean and Quinoa Wrap

Avocado and Egg Sandwich

Turkey and Spinach Sandwich

Chickpea Salad Sandwich

Berry Spinach Salad

Calories per Serving:
150

Fat: 10g

Protein: 3g

Carbohydrates: 14g

Prep Time: 10 minutes Serving Size: 4 servings

For the Salad:

6 cups fresh spinach leaves, washed and dried

1 cup fresh strawberries, sliced

1/2 cup fresh blueberries

1/2 cup fresh raspberries

1/4 cup red onion, thinly sliced

1/4 cup sliced almonds, optional, can be substituted with sunflower seeds for nut-free

1/4 cup crumbled feta cheese, optional, omit for dairy-free and vegan

For the Dressing:

2 tablespoons extra virgin olive oil

1 tablespoon balsamic vinegar

1 teaspoon honey or maple syrup for vegan

1 teaspoon Dijon mustard

Salt and pepper

Gluten-Free: Yes

Dairy-Free: Yes

Vegan: Yes

Nut-Free: No

1. In a large salad bowl, add the spinach, cut strawberries, blueberries, raspberries, and red onion. If using, add the sliced almonds and crumbled feta cheese.
2. In a small dish or container, mix together the olive oil, balsamic vinegar, honey, Dijon mustard, salt, and pepper until thoroughly blended.
3. Drizzle the dressing over the salad and gently toss to mix all the ingredients equally. Adjust the seasoning with extra salt and pepper if required.

4. Divide the salad into four portions and eat immediately.

For a Nut-Free Version, swap the almonds with sunflower seeds or pumpkin seeds, which still add a great crunch.

For a creamier dressing, you may add a tablespoon of tahini or avocado.

Turmeric Chickpea Salad

Calories per Serving:
220

Prep Time: 10 minutes Cooking Time: 5 minutes Serving Size: 4 servings

Fat: 9g

Protein: 7g

Carbohydrates: 28g

For the Chickpeas:

1 can (15 oz) chickpeas, drained and rinsed

1 tablespoon olive oil

1 teaspoon ground turmeric

1/2 teaspoon ground cumin

1/2 teaspoon smoked paprika

Gluten-Free: Yes

Salt and pepper

Dairy-Free: Yes

For the Salad:

Vegan: Yes

4 cups mixed greens

Nut-Free: Yes

1/2 red bell pepper, diced

1/2 cucumber, diced

1/4 red onion, thinly sliced

1/4 cup fresh cilantro or parsley, chopped

1 avocado, sliced or cubed

1/4 cup pumpkin seeds

For the Dressing:

2 tablespoons olive oil

1 tablespoon apple cider vinegar or lemon juice

1 teaspoon Dijon mustard

1/2 teaspoon ground turmeric

1/2 teaspoon honey or maple syrup

Salt and pepper

Prepare the Chickpeas:

1. Preheat a large skillet over medium heat.
2. In a bowl, mix the drained chickpeas with olive oil, turmeric, cumin, smoked paprika, salt, and pepper until well-coated.
3. Add the seasoned chickpeas to the pan and toast them for approximately 5 minutes, turning regularly, until they are somewhat crispy and golden brown. Set aside to cool.

Assemble the Salad:

4. In a large salad dish, combine the mixed greens, red bell pepper, cucumber, red onion, and fresh herbs (cilantro or parsley).
5. Add the roasted chickpeas and avocado to the salad.

6. Prepare the Dressing: In a small dish or container, mix together the olive oil, apple cider vinegar (or lemon juice), Dijon mustard, turmeric, honey (if using), salt, and pepper until thoroughly incorporated.

Toss and Serve:

7. Drizzle the dressing over the salad and toss lightly to mix.
8. Sprinkle with pumpkin seeds for extra texture, if preferred.

For extra protein, try topping the salad with grilled chicken or tofu.

Beet and Arugula Salad

Calories per Serving: 180

Fat: 12g

Protein: 4g

Carbohydrates: 16g

Prep Time: 10 minutes Cooking Time: 40 minutes Serving Size: 4 servings

4 medium beets, peeled and diced	1 tablespoon balsamic vinegar
4 cups fresh arugula	1 teaspoon Dijon mustard
1/4 cup walnuts, chopped	1 teaspoon maple syrup
1/4 red onion, thinly sliced	Salt and pepper
1/4 cup pomegranate seeds	
2 tablespoons extra-virgin olive oil	

Gluten-Free: Yes

Dairy-Free: Yes

Vegan: Yes

Nut-Free: Yes

1. Preheat your oven to 400°F (200°C). Place the chopped beets on a baking sheet lined with parchment paper. Drizzle with a little olive oil, salt, and pepper. Roast for 30-40 minutes, until soft. Allow them to cool somewhat.
2. In a large salad dish, add the fresh arugula. Top with the roasted beets, red onion slices, walnuts, and pomegranate seeds (if using).
3. In a small bowl, mix together the extra-virgin olive oil, balsamic vinegar, Dijon mustard, maple syrup (if using), salt, and pepper until thoroughly incorporated.
4. Drizzle the dressing over the salad and toss lightly to cover the contents evenly.
5. Divide the salad among four dishes and eat

Apple Walnut Salad

Calories per Serving: 220

Prep Time: 10 minutes Serving Size: 4 servings

Fat: 16g

Protein: 3g

Carbohydrates: 18g

4 cups mixed greens

2 medium apples, thinly sliced, use a variety like Granny Smith for tartness or Honeycrisp for sweetness

1/2 cup walnuts, toasted

1/4 cup dried cranberries

1/4 red onion, thinly sliced

1/4 cup pomegranate seeds

1/4 cup extra-virgin olive oil

2 tablespoons apple cider vinegar

1 teaspoon Dijon mustard

1 teaspoon honey or maple syrup

Salt and pepper

Gluten-Free: Yes

Dairy-Free: Yes

Vegan: Yes

Nut-Free: No

1. In a large bowl, combine the mixed greens, apple slices, toasted walnuts, dried cranberries, red onion, and pomegranate seeds if using.
2. In a small bowl, mix together the olive oil, apple cider vinegar, Dijon mustard, honey or maple syrup (if using), salt, and pepper until thoroughly blended.
3. Drizzle the dressing over the salad and toss gently until all components are uniformly covered.
4. Divide the salad among four dishes and serve

Chicken and Spinach Wrap

Calories per Serving: 320

Prep Time: 10 minutes Cooking Time: 15 minutes Serving Size: 2 servings

Fat: 12g

Protein: 30g

Carbohydrates: 24g

2 gluten-free wraps or whole grain wraps if not gluten-free

1 boneless, skinless chicken breast (6 oz)

1 cup fresh spinach leaves

Gluten-Free: Yes

1/2 avocado, sliced

Dairy-Free: Yes

1/4 red onion, thinly sliced

Nut-Free: Yes

1/2 cup cherry tomatoes, halved

1 tablespoon olive oil

1/2 teaspoon turmeric

1/2 teaspoon ground cumin

1/4 teaspoon paprika

Salt and pepper

1 tablespoon hummus

1. Season the chicken breast with turmeric, cumin, paprika, salt, and pepper. Heat the olive oil in a pan over medium heat.
2. Add the seasoned chicken breast to the pan and cook for approximately 6-7 minutes on each side, or until thoroughly done and no longer pink in the middle. Remove from heat and let it rest for a few minutes before slicing it into thin strips.
3. While the chicken is cooking, reheat the gluten-free wraps in a dry pan over medium heat for approximately 1-2 minutes on each side, or until they are flexible.
4. Spread a small amount of hummus (if using) on each wrap. Evenly arrange the spinach leaves, avocado slices, red onion, and cherry tomatoes over the wraps. Place the sliced chicken on top.

5. Fold the edges of each wrap inside and then roll it up securely from the bottom. Cut the wrap in half and serve immediately.

For added crunch, you might add some shredded carrots or cucumbers to the wrap.

Falafel Wrap

Calories per Serving:
350

Fat: 12g

Protein: 10g

Carbohydrates: 50g

Gluten-Free: Yes

Dairy-Free: Yes

Vegan: Yes

Nut-Free: Yes

Prep Time: 15 minutes **Cooking Time:** 20 minutes **Serving Size:** 4 wraps

For the Falafel:

1 1/2 cups cooked chickpeas or canned, drained and rinsed

1/2 small onion, roughly chopped

2 cloves garlic, minced

1/4 cup fresh parsley, chopped

1/4 cup fresh cilantro, chopped

2 tablespoons ground flaxseed or chickpea flour

1 teaspoon ground cumin

1 teaspoon ground coriander

1/2 teaspoon ground turmeric

1/2 teaspoon ground paprika

1/4 teaspoon ground black pepper

Salt to taste

2 tablespoons olive oil

For the Wrap:

4 gluten-free wraps or regular wraps if not gluten-sensitive

1 cup mixed greens

1/2 cup shredded red cabbage

1 medium cucumber, sliced

1 medium carrot, shredded

1/4 cup tahini sauce or hummus

1. In a food processor, blend the chickpeas, onion, garlic, parsley, cilantro, ground flaxseed, cumin, coriander, turmeric, paprika, black pepper, and salt. Pulse until the mixture is thoroughly blended but still somewhat lumpy. The mixture should hold together when pushed.
2. Using your hands, shape little balls or patties (approximately 2 teaspoons of ingredients per falafel). Flatten slightly to promote even cooking.
3. Heat the olive oil in a large pan over medium heat. Once heated, add the falafel patties, frying them for approximately 3-4 minutes on each side until golden brown and crispy. Remove from the skillet and put on a paper towel to drain excess oil.

Assemble the Wraps:

4. Lay out the gluten-free wraps. Spread a spoonful of tahini sauce or hummus in the middle of each wrap.
5. Add a layer of mixed greens, followed by shredded red cabbage, cucumber slices, and shredded carrot.
6. Place 3-4 falafel patties on top of the veggies.
7. Fold in the edges of the wrap and roll it up securely. Slice in half if preferred and serve immediately.

For added crunch, you may add sliced radishes or pickles to the wrap.

Black Bean and Quinoa Wrap

Calories per Serving: 350

Fat: 10g

Protein: 12g

Carbohydrates: 55g

Prep Time: 15 minutes Cooking Time: 20 minutes Serving Size: 4 wraps

Gluten-Free: Yes

Dairy-Free: Yes

Vegan: Yes

Nut-Free: Yes

For the Quinoa:

1/2 cup quinoa, rinsed

1 cup water or vegetable broth

For the Filling:

1 can (15 oz) black beans, drained and rinsed

1 cup corn kernels (fresh, frozen, or canned)

1/2 red bell pepper, diced

1/4 cup red onion, finely chopped

1 avocado, diced

1/4 cup fresh cilantro, chopped

Juice of 1 lime

1 teaspoon ground cumin

1/2 teaspoon smoked paprika

Salt and pepper

For the Wrap:

4 large gluten-free wraps or tortillas

1 cup baby spinach or mixed greens

1/4 cup dairy-free yogurt or hummus

Cook the Quinoa:

1. In a medium saucepan, bring the quinoa and water or vegetable broth to a boil.
2. Reduce the heat to low, cover, and simmer for approximately 15 minutes, or until the quinoa is cooked and the water is absorbed. Fluff with a fork and leave aside to cool somewhat.
3. Prepare the Filling: In a large mixing bowl, add the cooked quinoa, black beans, corn, red bell pepper, red onion, avocado, and cilantro. - Add lime juice, ground cumin, smoked paprika, salt, and pepper. Toss everything together until fully incorporated.

Assemble the Wraps:

4. Lay out the gluten-free wraps on a clean surface.
5. Spread a thin layer of dairy-free yogurt or hummus on each wrap if using.
6. Place a handful of baby spinach or mixed greens in the middle of each wrap.
7. Spoon a liberal quantity of the black bean and quinoa filling onto the leaves.

8. Wrap It Up: Fold in the edges of the wrap, then roll it up securely from the bottom. Slice each wrap in half if desired.

9. Serve: Serve the wraps immediately, or wrap them in foil for an on-the-go supper.

Ensure your wraps are gluten-free if required. There are several choices available, including ones made from brown rice, cassava, or other gluten-free grains.

Dairy-Free Yogurt or Hummus: This adds creaminess to the wrap, but it's optional. You may also add a dash of spicy sauce for added taste.

The filling may be prepared ahead of time and kept in the refrigerator for up to 3 days.

Avocado and Egg Sandwich

Calories per Serving: 350

Prep Time: 5 minutes Cooking Time: 5 minutes Serving Size: 1 sandwich

Fat: 24g

Protein: 13g

Carbohydrates: 28g

2 slices of gluten-free bread or regular bread if not gluten-sensitive

1/2 ripe avocado

1 large egg

1/4 teaspoon turmeric

1/4 teaspoon ground black pepper

1/4 teaspoon paprika

1 teaspoon extra-virgin olive oil or avocado oil

A pinch of sea salt

A few fresh spinach leaves

A squeeze of fresh lemon juice

Gluten-Free: Yes

Dairy-Free: Yes

Vegetarian: Yes

Nut-Free: Yes

1. Heat the olive oil in a small non-stick pan over medium heat. Crack the egg into the pan, sprinkle it with turmeric, black pepper, paprika, and a bit of salt. Cook until the white is set and the yolk is cooked to your taste (about 3 minutes for a runny yolk or 5 minutes for a firmer yolk). Remove from heat and put aside.

2. While the egg is cooking, split the avocado in half, remove the pit, and spoon the meat into a small dish. Mash the avocado with a fork until smooth. Add a bit of salt, black pepper, and a squeeze of lemon juice, if using.

3. Toast the pieces of gluten-free bread if preferred. Spread the mashed avocado equally on one piece of the bread. Top with the cooked egg and fresh spinach leaves, if using. Place the second piece of bread on top to finish the sandwich.

4. Cut the sandwich in half and eat immediately.

Turkey and Spinach Sandwich

Calories per Serving: 350

Fat: 12g

Protein: 25g

Carbohydrates: 36g

Prep Time: 10 minutes Serving Size: 1 sandwich

2 slices of whole-grain bread or gluten-free bread

3-4 ounces cooked turkey breast, thinly sliced

1/2 cup fresh spinach leaves

1/4 avocado, sliced

1 teaspoon Dijon mustard

1/4 teaspoon ground turmeric

1/4 teaspoon ground black pepper

1/4 teaspoon paprika

Gluten-Free:

Dairy-Free: Yes

1 small tomato, sliced

1 tablespoon hummus or dairy-free mayonnaise

1. If you wish, you may gently toast the bread pieces for a little crunch.
2. On one piece of bread, spread the hummus or dairy-free mayonnaise. If using, add the Dijon mustard.
3. Sprinkle the ground turmeric evenly over the spread. Add the ground black pepper and paprika to taste.
4. Layer the sliced turkey breast on the prepared bread. Add the fresh spinach leaves, avocado slices, and tomato slices.
5. Place the second piece of bread on top, push slightly, and cut the sandwich in two. Enjoy instantly.

To make this sandwich gluten-free, just use your favorite gluten-free bread.

For a dairy-free alternative, verify that the mayonnaise or spread used is free from dairy ingredients.

Chickpea Salad Sandwich

Calories per Serving: 320

Fat: 10g

Protein: 12g

Carbohydrates: 43g

Prep Time: 15 minutes Serving Size: 1 sandwich

1 can (15 oz) chickpeas, drained and rinsed

2 tablespoons vegan mayonnaise or plain Greek yogurt if not strictly vegan

1 tablespoon Dijon mustard

1 tablespoon lemon juice

1/4 cup finely chopped celery

1/4 cup finely chopped red bell pepper

1/4 cup finely chopped red onion

1 tablespoon chopped fresh parsley

1/2 teaspoon ground turmeric

1/4 teaspoon garlic powder

1/4 teaspoon paprika

Salt and pepper to taste

2 slices of gluten-free bread or regular whole grain bread, if not gluten-free

Leafy greens or lettuce for serving

Gluten-Free: Yes

Dairy-Free: Yes

Vegan: Yes

1. In a medium basin, mash the chickpeas using a fork or potato masher until largely broken down but still somewhat chunky.
2. Add the vegan mayonnaise, Dijon mustard, lemon juice, celery, red bell pepper, red onion, parsley (if using), turmeric, garlic powder, paprika, salt, and pepper. Mix until completely blended.
3. Spread the chickpea salad mixture equally over one piece of bread. Top with leafy greens or lettuce, then add the second piece of bread on top.
4. Cut the sandwich in half if preferred and serve

For a crisp texture, try adding thin slices of cucumber or radish.

CHAPTER 6
GRAINS AND LEGUMES

Brown Rice and Bean Burrito

Calories per Serving: 350

Fat: 8g

Protein: 14g

Carbohydrates: 60g

Prep Time: 10 minutes Cooking Time: 30 minutes Serving Size: 4 servings

Gluten-Free: Yes

Dairy-Free: Yes

Vegan: Yes

For the Bowl:

1 cup brown rice

1 can (15 oz) black beans, drained and rinsed

1 cup corn kernels (fresh, frozen, or canned)

1 red bell pepper, diced

1 cup cherry tomatoes, halved

1 avocado, diced

1/4 cup chopped fresh cilantro

Juice of 1 lime

For the Dressing:

2 tablespoons extra-virgin olive oil

1 tablespoon apple cider vinegar

1 teaspoon ground cumin

1/2 teaspoon smoked paprika

1/2 teaspoon garlic powder

1/4 teaspoon ground turmeric

Salt and pepper

1. Rinse the brown rice in cold water. In a medium pot, mix 1 cup of brown rice with 2 cups of water. Bring to a boil, then decrease the heat to low, cover, and simmer for approximately 30 minutes, or until the rice is cooked and the water is absorbed. Fluff with a fork and let it cool somewhat.
2. In a large bowl, mix the black beans, corn, sliced red bell pepper, cherry tomatoes, and chopped cilantro. Add the lime juice and stir to blend thoroughly.

3. In a small bowl, mix together the olive oil, apple cider vinegar, cumin, smoked paprika, garlic powder, turmeric, salt, and pepper.
4. Divide the cooked brown rice into 4 dishes. Top each bowl with the black bean and veggie mixture. Add chopped avocado on top of each bowl.
5. Drizzle the dressing over the bowls before serving.

Barley and Mushroom Risotto

Calories per Serving: 280

Fat: 6g

Protein: 8g

Carbohydrates: 45g

Prep Time: 10 minutes Cooking Time: 40 minutes Serving Size: 4 servings

1 cup pearled barley

2 tablespoons olive oil

1 medium onion, finely chopped

3 cloves garlic, minced

2 cups mushrooms, sliced, cremini or shiitake

1/2 cup dry white wine

4 cups vegetable broth

1 cup water more as needed

1/2 teaspoon dried thyme or 1 teaspoon fresh thyme

1/2 teaspoon dried rosemary or 1 teaspoon fresh rosemary

1/2 teaspoon turmeric

1/4 cup nutritional yeast

Salt and black pepper

Gluten-Free: No

Dairy-Free: Yes

Vegan: Yes

1. Rinse the pearled barley under cold water and leave aside.
2. Heat olive oil in a large pan over medium heat. Add the chopped onion and simmer until transparent, approximately 5 minutes. Add the minced garlic and simmer for another 1-2 minutes until fragrant.
3. Add the sliced mushrooms to the pan and sauté until they are browned and soft, approximately 8-10 minutes.
4. Stir in the rinsed barley and simmer for 1-2 minutes. If using, pour in the white wine and simmer until it is largely absorbed.
5. Add 1 cup of vegetable broth and mix until it is largely absorbed. Continue adding the broth, one cup at a time, allowing it to be absorbed before adding the next cup. Stir

regularly. You may also add water if the mixture gets too thick.

6. When the barley is soft and creamy (after around 30-40 minutes), toss in the thyme, rosemary, turmeric, and nutritional yeast if using. Season with salt and black pepper to taste.

7. Once the risotto has acquired a creamy consistency, remove from heat and serve warm.

Red Lentil Curry

Calories per Serving: 250

Fat: 8g

Protein: 13g

Carbohydrates: 35g

Prep Time: 10 minutes Cooking Time: 30 minutes Serving Size: 4 servings

1 cup red lentils, rinsed and drained

1 tablespoon coconut oil or olive oil

1 medium onion, chopped

3 garlic cloves, minced

1 tablespoon fresh ginger, minced

1 can (14.5 oz) diced tomatoes

1 cup coconut milk (unsweetened)

2 cups vegetable broth (low sodium)

1 tablespoon curry powder

1 teaspoon ground turmeric

1 teaspoon ground cumin

1/2 teaspoon paprika

1/2 teaspoon ground coriander

1/2 teaspoon black pepper

1/2 teaspoon sea salt or to taste

1 cup spinach

Gluten-Free: Yes

Dairy-Free: Yes

Vegan: Yes

1. In a big saucepan, heat the coconut oil over medium heat. Add the chopped onion and simmer until transparent, approximately 5 minutes. Add the minced garlic and ginger, and simmer for another 1-2 minutes until fragrant.
2. Stir in the curry powder, turmeric, cumin, paprika, coriander, black pepper, and salt. Cook for around 1 minute to toast the seasonings.
3. Add the chopped tomatoes, coconut milk, and vegetable broth to the saucepan. Stir well to mix.
4. Add the washed red lentils. Bring the mixture to a boil, then decrease the heat to low and cover. Simmer for around 20-25

minutes, or until the lentils are soft and the curry has thickened. Stir periodically to avoid sticking.

5. If using, toss in the spinach until wilted. Adjust seasoning to taste if required. Serve hot over rice or with a side of naan.

Millet and Vegetable Stir-Fry

Calories per Serving: 250

Fat: 7g

Protein: 8g

Carbohydrates: 35g

Prep Time: 15 minutes Cooking Time: 20 minutes Serving Size: 4 servings

Gluten-Free: Yes

Dairy-Free: Yes

Vegan: Yes

1 cup millet

2 cups water or vegetable broth

1 tablespoon olive oil (or avocado oil)

1 medium onion, diced

2 cloves garlic, minced

1 bell pepper, sliced

1 medium zucchini, sliced

1 cup broccoli florets

1 cup snap peas

1 medium carrot, julienned

2 tablespoons tamari (gluten-free soy sauce) or coconut aminos

1 tablespoon fresh ginger, grated

1/2 teaspoon ground turmeric

1/2 teaspoon ground black pepper

1 tablespoon sesame seeds

Fresh cilantro or green onions

1. Rinse the millet under cold water. In a medium saucepan, mix the millet and water or vegetable broth. Bring to a boil, then decrease heat to low, cover, and simmer for approximately 15 minutes, or until the liquid is absorbed and the millet is soft. Remove from heat and let it rest covered for 5 minutes, then fluff with a fork.

2. While the millet is cooking, heat the olive oil in a large pan or wok over medium-high heat. Add the diced onion and simmer for 3-4 minutes until softened.

3. Add the minced garlic and heat for a further minute. Then, add the bell pepper, zucchini, broccoli, snap peas, and carrot. Stir-fry the veggies for approximately 5-7 minutes, or until they are crisp-tender.

4. Add the tamari or coconut aminos, grated ginger, crushed turmeric, and black pepper to the veggies. Stir well to coat the veggies evenly with the spices.

5. Add the cooked millet to the pan with the veggies. Stir well to incorporate and cook through, approximately 2-3 minutes.

6. Garnish with sesame seeds and fresh cilantro or green onions if preferred. Serve warm.

For extra crunch, you may also add a handful of roasted nuts or seeds..

Chickpea and Spinach Curry

Calories per Serving: 300

Fat: 10g

Protein: 12g

Carbohydrates: 40g

Prep Time: 10 minutes Cooking Time: 20 minutes Serving Size: 4 servings

1 tablespoon olive oil

1 medium onion, finely chopped

3 garlic cloves, minced

1 tablespoon fresh ginger, minced

1 teaspoon ground turmeric

1 teaspoon ground cumin

Gluten-Free: Yes

1 teaspoon ground coriander

Dairy-Free: Yes

1/2 teaspoon paprika

Vegan: Yes

1/2 teaspoon cayenne pepper

1 can (15 oz) chickpeas, drained and rinsed

1 can (14.5 oz) diced tomatoes (no added sugar)

1 cup vegetable broth

4 cups fresh spinach, washed and chopped

1/2 cup coconut milk (canned)

Salt and pepper

1 tablespoon fresh lemon juice

1. Heat olive oil in a large pan over medium heat. Add the chopped onion and simmer until transparent, approximately 5 minutes. Add the minced garlic and ginger, simmering for another 1-2 minutes until fragrant.
2. Stir in the ground turmeric, cumin, coriander, paprika, and cayenne pepper (if using). Cook for 1 minute to toast the seasonings.
3. Add the drained chickpeas, diced tomatoes, and vegetable broth. Stir to incorporate and bring to a simmer. Reduce heat and let it simmer for approximately 10 minutes to enable the flavors to mingle.

4. Stir in the chopped spinach and coconut milk. Cook for another 2-3 minutes until the spinach is wilted and the curry is cooked through.
5. Season with salt and pepper to taste. If preferred, add a tablespoon of fresh lemon juice for added taste. Serve hot over rice or with gluten-free naan.

The cayenne pepper provides spice but may be eliminated if you want a milder curry.

Quinoa and Sweet Potato Chili

Calories per Serving: 300

Fat: 7g

Protein: 11g

Carbohydrates: 49g

Prep Time: 15 minutes Cooking Time: 35 minutes Serving Size: 4 servings

1 tablespoon olive oil

1 large onion, diced

2 cloves garlic, minced

1 large bell pepper, diced

2 medium sweet potatoes, peeled and diced

1 cup quinoa, rinsed

1 can (14.5 oz) diced tomatoes (no salt added)

1 can (15 oz) black beans, drained and rinsed

1 can (15 oz) kidney beans, drained and rinsed

1 cup vegetable broth (low sodium)

1 tablespoon ground cumin

1 tablespoon smoked paprika

1 teaspoon ground turmeric

1/2 teaspoon ground chili powder

Salt and pepper

1 cup frozen corn

1/4 cup chopped fresh cilantro

Gluten-Free: Yes

Dairy-Free: Yes

Vegan: Yes

1. Heat olive oil in a big saucepan over medium heat. Add the chopped onion and sauté until transparent, approximately 5 minutes. Add minced garlic and simmer for another 1-2 minutes until fragrant.
2. Stir in the chopped bell pepper and sweet potatoes. Cook for approximately 5 minutes, stirring periodically.
3. Add the rinsed quinoa, chopped tomatoes, black beans, kidney beans, vegetable broth, cumin, smoked paprika, turmeric, chili powder, salt, and pepper. Stir well to mix.
4. Bring the mixture to a boil, then decrease the heat to low. Cover and let it boil for 20-25 minutes, or until the sweet potatoes are soft and the quinoa is cooked. If using frozen corn, mix it in during the final 5 minutes of cooking.
5. Taste the chili and adjust seasoning if required. Garnish with fresh cilantro if desired.

Ladle the chili into bowls and serve hot.

Wild Rice and Cranberry Salad

Calories per Serving: 220

Fat: 7g

Protein: 6g

Carbohydrates: 32g

Prep Time: 15 minutes Cooking Time: 35 minutes Serving Size: 4 servings

1 cup wild rice

2 1/2 cups water or vegetable broth

1/2 cup dried cranberries

1/4 cup chopped walnuts or pecans

1/4 cup finely chopped red onion

1/2 cup diced celery

1/2 cup diced apple

2 tablespoons olive oil

1 tablespoon apple cider vinegar

1 tablespoon fresh lemon juice

1 teaspoon Dijon mustard

1/2 teaspoon dried thyme

Salt and pepper

Gluten-Free: Yes

Dairy-Free: Yes

Vegan: Yes

1. Rinse the wild rice under cold water. In a medium saucepan, bring 2 1/2 cups water or vegetable broth to a boil. Add the wild rice, lower heat to low, cover, and simmer for approximately 35 minutes, or until the rice is soft but chewy. Drain any extra liquid and allow the rice cool to room temperature
2. \While the rice is cooking, cut the red onion, celery, and apple (if using). Toast the walnuts in a dry pan over medium heat for 5 minutes or until aromatic, then let them cool.
3. In a small bowl, mix together the olive oil, apple cider vinegar, lemon juice, Dijon mustard, dried thyme, salt, and pepper.
4. In a large bowl, mix the cooked wild rice, dried cranberries, chopped walnuts, red onion, celery, and apple. Pour the dressing over the salad and toss to coat evenly.

5. Let the salad rest in the refrigerator for at least 30 minutes to enable the flavors to mingle. Toss again before serving.

Black Bean and Corn Salad

Calories per Serving: 220

Fat: 6g

Protein: 8g

Carbohydrates: 33g

Prep Time: 15 minutes Serving Size: 4 servings

1 can (15 oz) black beans, drained and rinsed

1 cup fresh or frozen corn kernels (if frozen, thawed)

1 red bell pepper, diced

1 cup cherry tomatoes, halved

1/4 cup red onion, finely chopped

1/4 cup fresh cilantro, chopped

1 avocado, diced

2 tablespoons extra-virgin olive oil

Juice of 1 lime

1/2 teaspoon ground cumin

1/2 teaspoon smoked paprika

Salt and pepper

Gluten-Free: Yes

Dairy-Free: Yes

Vegan: Yes

1. Drain and rinse the black beans. If using frozen corn, defrost it by putting it in a basin of water or running it under cold water.
2. In a large bowl, add the black beans, corn, diced red bell pepper, cherry tomatoes, red onion, and chopped cilantro.
3. In a small bowl, mix together the olive oil, lime juice, ground cumin, smoked paprika, salt, and pepper.
4. Pour the dressing over the salad and toss lightly to mix. Add the diced avocado and mix gently to prevent mashing the avocado.
5. Let the salad rest for approximately 10 minutes to enable the flavors to mingle. Serve refrigerated or at room temperature.

Bulgur Wheat and Chickpea Salad

Calories per Serving: 250

Fat: 7g

Protein: 9g

Carbohydrates: 36g

Prep Time: 15 minutes Cooking Time: 10 minutes Serving Size: 4 servings

1 cup bulgur wheat

1 1/2 cups water or vegetable broth

1 can (15 oz) chickpeas, drained and rinsed

1 cup cherry tomatoes, halved

1 cucumber, diced

1/4 cup red onion, finely chopped

1/4 cup fresh mint, chopped

1/4 cup extra virgin olive oil

Juice of 1 lemon

1/2 teaspoon ground turmeric

1/2 teaspoon ground cumin

Salt and pepper

1/4 cup fresh parsley, chopped

Gluten-Free: No

Dairy-Free: Yes

Vegan: Yes

1. In a medium saucepan, bring 1 1/2 cups of water or vegetable broth to a boil. Add the bulgur wheat, decrease heat to low, cover, and simmer for 10 minutes until the liquid is absorbed and the bulgur is soft. Remove from heat and allow it to cool to room temperature.
2. While the bulgur is cooking, cut the cherry tomatoes, cucumber, red onion, parsley, and mint.
3. In a large bowl, mix the cooked bulgur wheat, chickpeas, cherry tomatoes, cucumber, red onion, parsley, and mint.
4. In a small bowl, mix together the olive oil, lemon juice, turmeric, cumin, salt, and pepper.
5. Pour the dressing over the salad and mix until all ingredients are well-coated. Adjust seasoning with extra salt and pepper if required.
6. Let the salad rest for at least 15 minutes to enable flavors to blend. Serve refrigerated or at room temperature.

Bulgur Wheat includes gluten, thus this dish is not ideal for persons with food intolerance. You may replace quinoa or rice for a gluten-free alternative.

Quinoa and Black Bean Tacos

Calories per Serving: 350

Fat: 8g

Protein: 14g

Carbohydrates: 55g

Gluten-Free: Yes

Dairy-Free: Yes

Vegan: Yes

Prep Time: 15 minutes Cooking Time: 20 minutes Serving Size: 4 tacos

For the Quinoa and Black Bean Filling:

1 cup quinoa, rinsed

2 cups water

1 can (15 oz) black beans, drained and rinsed

1 tablespoon olive oil

1 small onion, diced

2 cloves garlic, minced

1 red bell pepper, diced

1 cup corn kernels (fresh, frozen, or canned)

1 teaspoon ground cumin

1/2 teaspoon smoked paprika

1/2 teaspoon chili powder

1/2 teaspoon turmeric

Salt and pepper

For Serving:

4 gluten-free taco shells or tortillas

1 avocado, sliced

1 cup shredded lettuce

1/2 cup cherry tomatoes, halved

Fresh cilantro leaves, chopped

Lime wedges

1. In a medium saucepan, bring 2 cups of water to a boil. Add the rinsed quinoa, lower heat to low, cover, and simmer for approximately 15 minutes, or until the quinoa is cooked and the water is absorbed. Fluff with a fork and put aside.
2. While the quinoa cooks, heat olive oil in a large pan over medium heat. Add the chopped onion and sauté until transparent, approximately 5 minutes. Add the minced garlic and simmer for another 1 minute.
3. Stir in the diced red bell pepper and simmer for 3 minutes. Add the corn, cooked quinoa, black beans, cumin, smoked paprika, chili powder, and turmeric. Cook for another 5-7 minutes, stirring periodically, until cooked through and thoroughly mixed. Season with salt and pepper to taste.
4. Warm the gluten-free taco shells or tortillas according to package directions. Divide the quinoa and black bean mixture equally among the taco shells.

Top each taco with sliced avocado, shredded lettuce, cherry tomatoes, and chopped cilantro, if using. Serve with lime wedges on the side.

CHAPTER 7

SOUPS AND STEWS

Turmeric Chicken Soup

Lentil and Spinach Soup

Miso Soup with Tofu

Kale and White Bean Soup

Quinoa Vegetable Soup

Beet and Ginger Soup

Broccoli and Spinach Soup

Spicy Chickpea Stew

Mushroom and Barley Soup

Pea and Mint Soup

Turmeric Chicken Soup

Calories per Serving: 250

Fat: 7g

Protein: 30g

Carbohydrates: 15g

Prep Time: 15 minutes Cooking Time: 30 minutes Serving Size: 4 servings

Gluten-Free: Yes

Dairy-Free: Yes

Low-Carb: Yes

2 tablespoons olive oil

1 medium onion, diced

3 cloves garlic, minced

1 tablespoon fresh ginger, grated

1 tablespoon ground turmeric

1/2 teaspoon ground cumin

1/2 teaspoon ground coriander

4 cups chicken broth (make sure it's gluten-free)

2 cups cooked, shredded chicken preferably from a rotisserie chicken or pre-cooked

1 cup chopped carrots about 2 medium carrots

1 cup chopped celery about 2 stalks

1 cup baby spinach or kale

1 tablespoon lemon juice

Salt and pepper

1. Heat the olive oil in a big saucepan over medium heat. Add the chopped onion and sauté until transparent, approximately 5 minutes. Add the minced garlic and grated ginger, and sauté for another 2 minutes.
2. Stir in the ground turmeric, cumin, and coriander. Cook for 1 minute until the spices are aromatic.
3. Pour in the chicken broth and bring to a boil. Add the diced carrots and celery. Reduce heat to a simmer and cook until the veggies are soft, approximately 10 minutes.
4. Stir in the shredded chicken and baby spinach (or kale). Simmer for another 5 minutes until the spinach has wilted and the chicken is cooked through.

5. Add lemon juice if using, and season with salt and pepper to taste. Serve hot.

Lentil and Spinach Soup

**Calories per Serving:
220**

Fat: 3g

Protein: 13g

Carbohydrates: 35g

**Prep Time: 10 minutes Cooking Time: 30 minutes Serving Size: 4
servings**

1 tablespoon olive oil

1 medium onion, diced

2 cloves garlic, minced

1 large carrot, diced

2 celery stalks, diced

1 cup dried green or brown lentils,
rinsed and drained

1 can (14.5 oz) diced tomatoes (no
salt added)

6 cups vegetable broth

2 cups fresh spinach leaves,
chopped

1 teaspoon ground turmeric

1 teaspoon ground cumin

1/2 teaspoon smoked paprika

Salt and pepper

1 tablespoon lemon juice

Gluten-Free: Yes

Dairy-Free: Yes

Vegan: Yes

1. In a large saucepan, heat the olive oil over medium heat. Add
    the chopped onion and simmer for 3-4 minutes until
    transparent
2. Add the garlic, carrot, and celery to the saucepan. Cook for a
    further 5 minutes until the veggies begin to soften. Stir in the
    ground turmeric, cumin, and smoked paprika.
3. Add the rinsed lentils, diced tomatoes, and vegetable broth.
    Bring the mixture to a boil, then decrease the heat to low.
    Simmer for 20-25 minutes, or until the lentils are soft.
4. Stir in the chopped spinach and simmer for a further 5
    minutes until the spinach is wilted.

5. **Season the soup with salt and pepper to taste. If preferred, add a tablespoon of lemon juice for added brightness. Serve hot.**

Miso Soup with Tofu

Calories per Serving: 120

Fat: 6g

Protein: 8g

Carbohydrates: 9g

Gluten-Free: Yes

Dairy-Free: Yes

Vegan: Yes

Prep Time: 10 minutes Cooking Time: 10 minutes Serving Size: 2 servings

4 cups water

1/4 cup gluten-free miso paste (white or yellow)

1 cup firm tofu, cubed

1/4 cup dried seaweed (wakame or nori)

2 green onions, sliced

1 small carrot, thinly sliced

1 tablespoon fresh ginger, grated

1 teaspoon sesame oil

1. If using dried seaweed, soak it in water for approximately 5 minutes until it softens. Drain and put aside.
2. In a medium saucepan, bring 4 cups of water to a simmer over medium heat. If using ginger, add it to the stew and boil for a few minutes to absorb the flavor.
3. Reduce the heat to low. In a small dish, dissolve the miso paste in a little quantity of boiling water (approximately 1/2 cup) until smooth. Stir this mixture into the saucepan with the simmering water. Avoid boiling the soup after adding miso to retain its helpful microbes.

4. Add the diced tofu and soaking seaweed to the saucepan. Simmer gently for approximately 5 minutes to cook the tofu and allow the flavors to mingle.
5. If using, add the sliced carrots and let them simmer for another 2-3 minutes until soft. Stir in the cut green onions and, if preferred, sesame oil.
6. Ladle the soup into bowls and enjoy the heat.

Kale and White Bean Soup

Calories per Serving:
220

Fat: 6g

Protein: 10g

Carbohydrates: 32g

Prep Time: 15 minutes Cooking Time: 30 minutes Serving Size: 4 servings

1A pair of about 8 ounce ribeye steaks

Four big eggs

1 tablespoon of beef tallow or butter

Pepper and salt

Gluten-Free: Yes

Dairy-Free: Yes

Vegan: Yes

Remove the steaks from the refrigerator and let them sit for about half an hour to come to room temperature. This guarantees uniform cooking..

Lightly season the steaks on both sides with salt and pepper.r.

Turn up the heat to high and thoroughly heat the cast iron skillet. Prior to adding the meat, the pan should be slightly smoking.

Quinoa Vegetable Soup

Calories per Serving: 220

Fat: 6g

Protein: 8g

Carbohydrates: 35g

Prep Time: 15 minutes Cooking Time: 30 minutes Serving Size: 4 servings

1 tablespoon olive oil

1 medium onion, diced

2 cloves garlic, minced

2 medium carrots, peeled and diced

2 celery stalks, diced

1 cup quinoa, rinsed

1 cup diced tomatoes (fresh or canned)

4 cups vegetable broth (ensure it's gluten-free)

1 cup chopped kale or spinach

1 cup sliced mushrooms

1 cup seaweed (wakame or nori), rehydrated and chopped

1 teaspoon dried thyme

1 teaspoon dried oregano

1/2 teaspoon turmeric

Salt and pepper

Gluten-Free: Yes

Dairy-Free: Yes

Vegan: Yes

Nut-Free: Yes

1. Dice the onion, carrots, celery, and mushrooms. Mince the garlic.
2. In a large saucepan, heat the olive oil over medium heat. Add the onion and garlic and sauté until transparent, approximately 3-4 minutes.
3. Add the carrots, celery, and mushrooms to the saucepan. Cook for a further 5 minutes, stirring occasionally.
4. Stir in the quinoa and chopped tomatoes. Cook for 2 minutes.
5. Pour in the veggie broth and add the dried thyme, oregano, and turmeric (if using). Bring to a boil.
6. Reduce heat to low, cover, and simmer for 15 minutes, or until the quinoa and veggies are cooked.

7. Stir in the chopped kale or spinach and rehydrated seaweed. Cook for a further 5 minutes until the greens are wilted and the seaweed is cooked through.
8. Season with salt and pepper to taste. Serve hot

Beet and Ginger Soup

Calories per Serving: 140

Fat: 4g

Protein: 3g

Carbohydrates: 23g

Prep Time: 15 minutes Cooking Time: 35 minutes Serving Size: 4 servings

4 medium beets, peeled and diced

1 tablespoon fresh ginger, peeled and minced (or 1 teaspoon ground ginger)

1 medium onion, chopped

2 cloves garlic, minced

1 tablespoon olive oil

4 cups vegetable broth

1 medium carrot, peeled and diced

1 small apple, peeled, cored, and diced

1 tablespoon lemon juice

Salt and pepper

Fresh parsley or cilantro

Gluten-Free: Yes

Dairy-Free: Yes

Vegan: Yes

Nut-Free: Yes

1. Peel and dice the beets and carrot, and cut the onion. Mince the garlic and ginger.
2. Heat olive oil in a big saucepan over medium heat. Add the onion and sauté until transparent, approximately 5 minutes. Add the garlic and ginger, simmering for another 1-2 minutes until fragrant.
3. Stir in the chopped beets and carrots. Cook for 5 minutes, stirring periodically.
4. Pour in the veggie broth and add the diced apple. Bring the mixture to a boil, then decrease the heat to low and allow it simmer for 30 minutes, or until the beets and carrots are soft.
5. Use an immersion blender to purée the soup until smooth. Alternatively, transfer the soup in stages to a blender and process until smooth. Return the pureed soup to the pot

6. Stir in lemon juice, and season with salt and pepper to taste. Garnish with fresh parsley or cilantro if preferred. Serve hot.
7. If you want a thicker soup, mix in part of the beets and carrots before adding all of the liquid.
8. For a touch of added richness, you may whisk in a splash of coconut milk at the end.

Broccoli and Spinach Soup

**Calories per Serving:
120**

Prep Time: 10 minutes Cooking Time: 20 minutes Serving Size: 4 servings

Fat: 4g

Protein: 5g

Carbohydrates: 20g

2 tablespoons olive oil

4 cups vegetable broth

1 medium onion, chopped

1/2 teaspoon ground turmeric

3 cloves garlic, minced

1/2 teaspoon ground black pepper

1 large head broccoli, cut into florets

1/4 teaspoon ground cumin

2 cups fresh spinach

Salt (optional)

1 medium potato, peeled and diced

Gluten-Free: Yes

Dairy-Free: Yes

Vegan: Yes

Nut-Free: Yes

1. Wash and cut the broccoli, onion, garlic, and spinach. Dice the potato if using.
2. Heat olive oil in a big saucepan over medium heat. Add the chopped onion and garlic, and sauté until the onion is transparent, approximately 5 minutes.
3. Add the broccoli florets, diced potato (if using), and vegetable broth to the saucepan. Bring to a boil, then decrease heat and simmer for 10-15 minutes, or until the veggies are soft.
4. Stir in the fresh spinach, turmeric, black pepper, and cumin (if using). Cook for a further 2-3 minutes, or until the spinach is wilted.
5. Use an immersion blender to mix the soup until smooth. Alternatively, gently transfer the soup in stages to a tabletop blender and mix until smooth. If the soup is too thick, add a bit more vegetable broth to obtain the required consistency.
6. Adjust seasoning with salt if required. Serve hot.

7. Potatoes assist to thicken the soup and provide creaminess without adding dairy. You may eliminate it for a lighter version.
8. Immersion Blender is helpful for mixing soups right in the pot, minimizing cleaning time.

Spicy Chickpea Stew

Calories per Serving: 250

Fat: 7g

Protein: 11g

Carbohydrates: 35g

Prep Time: 15 minutes Cooking Time: 30 minutes Serving Size: 4 servings

1 tablespoon olive oil

1 large onion, diced

3 cloves garlic, minced

1 bell pepper, diced (red or yellow for sweetness)

1 can (15 oz) diced tomatoes

1 can (15 oz) chickpeas, drained and rinsed

1 cup vegetable broth or water

1 medium sweet potato, peeled and diced

1 teaspoon ground turmeric

1/2 teaspoon ground cumin

1/2 teaspoon smoked paprika

1/4 teaspoon cayenne pepper

1 teaspoon dried oregano

1/2 teaspoon black pepper

Salt to taste

2 cups fresh spinach or kale

Gluten-Free: Yes

Dairy-Free: Yes

Vegan: Yes

Nut-Free: Yes

1. Heat the olive oil in a big saucepan over medium heat. Add the chopped onion and sauté until transparent, approximately 5 minutes. Add the minced garlic and bell pepper, cooking for an additional 3 minutes until softened.
2. Stir in the ground turmeric, cumin, smoked paprika, cayenne pepper, oregano, black pepper, and salt. Cook for 1 minute until aromatic.
3. Add the diced tomatoes, chickpeas, vegetable broth, and sweet potato to the saucepan. Stir well to mix.

4. Bring the mixture to a boil, then decrease the heat to low. Cover and boil for 20 minutes, or until the sweet potatoes are soft and cooked through.
5. If using spinach or kale, mix it in during the final 5 minutes of simmering, allowing it to wilt and blend into the stew.
6. Ladle the stew into dishes and enjoy the heat.

Mushroom and Barley Soup

Calories per Serving:
220

Fat: 5g

Protein: 8g

Carbohydrates: 35g

Prep Time: 15 minutes **Cooking Time:** 45 minutes **Serving Size:** 4 servings

1 tablespoon olive oil

1 medium onion, diced

2 cloves garlic, minced

2 cups mushrooms , sliced

1 cup pearl barley

4 cups vegetable broth

Gluten-Free: No

2 medium carrots, diced

Dairy-Free: Yes

2 celery stalks, diced

Vegan: Yes

1 teaspoon dried thyme

1 teaspoon dried rosemary

1/2 teaspoon turmeric

1/4 teaspoon black pepper

1 cup spinach or kale, chopped

1 tablespoon lemon juice

1. In a large saucepan, heat the olive oil over medium heat.
2. Add the diced onion and garlic, and sauté until softened, approximately 5 minutes. Add the mushrooms and simmer until they release their moisture and start to brown, approximately 7 minutes.
3. Stir in the barley, vegetable broth, carrots, celery, thyme, rosemary, turmeric, and black pepper. Bring the mixture to a boil.
4. Reduce the heat to low, cover, and allow the soup simmer for 30 minutes, or until the barley is soft.

5. If using spinach or kale, toss it in during the final 5 minutes of simmering until wilted.
6. Stir in the lemon juice, if using, and adjust seasoning as required. Serve hot.
7. To make the soup gluten-free, replace the barley with quinoa, rice, or gluten-free pasta.

Lemon Juice gives a fresh note that may help balance the tastes, particularly if you enjoy a little acidity in your soups.

Pea and Mint Soup

Calories per Serving: 120

Prep Time: 10 minutes Cooking Time: 20 minutes Serving Size: 4 servings

Fat: 3g

Protein: 5g

Carbohydrates: 20g

2 cups frozen peas or fresh peas, if available	1/2 cup fresh mint leaves, chopped
1 tablespoon olive oil	1 teaspoon dried thyme
1 medium onion, chopped	Salt and pepper
2 garlic cloves, minced	1 tablespoon lemon juice
1 medium potato, peeled and diced	
4 cups vegetable broth (low sodium)	

Gluten-Free: Yes

Dairy-Free: Yes

Vegan: Yes

Nut-Free: Yes

1. Chop the onion and mince the garlic. Peel and dice the potato. If using fresh peas, shell them and leave aside.
2. In a large saucepan, heat the olive oil over medium heat. Add the diced onion and sauté for approximately 5 minutes until softened and transparent. Add the minced garlic and simmer for an additional 1-2 minutes until fragrant.
3. Add the diced potato and simmer for 5 minutes, stirring regularly. Add the frozen peas and veggie broth. Bring the mixture to a boil, then decrease the heat and simmer for 10-15 minutes, until the potato is soft and the peas are cooked through.
4. Using an immersion blender, mix the soup directly in the pot until smooth. Alternatively, transfer the soup in stages to a normal blender and mix until smooth. If the soup is too thick, add a little more vegetable broth or water to obtain your preferred consistency.

5. Stir in the chopped mint leaves and season with salt, pepper, and dry thyme (if using). Simmer for another 2 minutes to allow the flavors to mingle.
6. Ladle the soup into bowls. If preferred, add a dash of lemon juice for added brightness.

CHAPTER 8

SEAFOOD, MEAT AND PROTEIN

Turmeric Shrimp Stir-Fry

Mackerel with Lemon

Cod with Tomato Basil Sauce

Garlic Butter Shrimp

Seafood Paella

Turmeric Chicken and Vegetables

Ginger Beef Stir-Fry

Lemon Herb Chicken

Turkey and Potato Skillet

Rosemary Garlic Lamb Chops

Turmeric Shrimp Stir-Fry

**Calories per Serving:
280**

Fat: 10g

Protein: 28g

Carbohydrates: 18g

**Prep Time: 15 minutes Cooking Time: 10 minutes Serving Size: 2
servings**

12 oz (340g) large shrimp, peeled and deveined

1 tablespoon olive oil or avocado oil

1 bell pepper, sliced

1 cup snap peas

Gluten-Free: Yes

1 small carrot, thinly sliced

1 cup broccoli florets

Dairy-Free: Yes

Vegan: No

1 tablespoon fresh turmeric, grated or 1 teaspoon ground turmeric

1 tablespoon fresh ginger, grated

2 cloves garlic, minced

2 tablespoons coconut aminos or low-sodium soy sauce if not strictly gluten-free

1 tablespoon lemon juice or lime juice

1 teaspoon sesame seeds

1 green onion, sliced

1. Thaw the shrimp if frozen and pat dry. Slice veggies and prepare the turmeric, ginger, and garlic.
2. In a large skillet or wok, heat the olive oil over medium-high heat.
3. Add the shrimp to the pan and cook for 2-3 minutes on each side until they become pink and opaque. Remove shrimp from the pan and put aside.
4. In the same pan, add the bell pepper, snap peas, carrot, and broccoli. Stir-fry for 4-5 minutes until the veggies are tender-crisp.
5. Add the grated turmeric, ginger, and chopped garlic to the skillet. Stir and heat for another 1-2 minutes until aromatic.

6. Return the cooked shrimp to the skillet. Add the coconut aminos and lemon juice, stirring to coat everything evenly. Cook for another 1-2 minutes until cooked through.
7. Garnish with sesame seeds and green onions if preferred. Serve immediately.

Coconut Aminos is a gluten-free alternative to soy sauce, delivering a slightly sweeter taste. If you're not completely avoiding gluten, low-sodium soy sauce is also an option.

You may add a sprinkle of cayenne pepper if you prefer more heat.

Mackerel with Lemon

Calories per Serving:
320

Fat: 22g

Protein: 28g

Carbohydrates: 2g

Prep Time: 10 minutes Cooking Time: 15-20 minutes Serving Size: 2 servings

2 mackerel filets (about 6 oz each)

1 lemon, thinly sliced

2 tablespoons olive oil

2 garlic cloves, minced

1 tablespoon fresh parsley, chopped or 1 teaspoon dried parsley

1 tablespoon fresh dill, chopped or 1 teaspoon dried dill

1 teaspoon dried oregano

Salt and pepper

Gluten-Free: Yes

Dairy-Free: Yes

Vegan: No

Nut-Free: Yes

1. Preheat your oven to 375°F (190°C).
2. Rinse the mackerel filets under cold water and wipe them dry with paper towels. Place them on a baking sheet lined with parchment paper.
3. Drizzle the olive oil over the filets. Sprinkle the minced garlic, parsley, dill, oregano, salt, and pepper equally over the filets. Place the lemon slices on top of the filets.
4. Bake the mackerel in the preheated oven for 15-20 minutes, or until the fish is opaque and flakes readily with a fork.
5. Remove from the oven and let it rest for a few minutes before serving. Serve with more lemon wedges if desired.

Cod with Tomato Basil Sauce

**Calories per Serving:
250**

Fat: 8g

Protein: 32g

Carbohydrates: 12g

**Prep Time: 10 minutes Cooking Time: 20 minutes Serving Size: 4
servings**

4 cod filets (6 oz each)

1 tablespoon olive oil

1 medium onion, finely chopped

2 cloves garlic, minced

1 can (14.5 oz) diced tomatoes (no
salt added)

1/4 cup tomato paste

1/2 cup water or vegetable
broth

1 tablespoon fresh basil,
chopped or 1 teaspoon dried
basil

1/2 teaspoon dried oregano

1/4 teaspoon red pepper flakes

Salt and black pepper

Gluten-Free: Yes

Dairy-Free: Yes

Paleo: Yes

1. Preheat your oven to 375°F (190°C).
2. In a medium saucepan, heat olive oil over medium heat. Add
   the chopped onion and simmer until transparent,
   approximately 5 minutes. Add the minced garlic and simmer
   for another minute.
3. Stir in the chopped tomatoes, tomato paste, and water or
   broth. Add the fresh basil, oregano, red pepper flakes (if
   using), and salt and pepper to taste. Simmer the sauce for
   approximately 10 minutes, until it thickens slightly.
4. While the sauce is boiling, season the cod filets with salt and
   black pepper. Place them in a baking dish.
5. Pour the tomato basil sauce over the cod filets, ensuring they
   are completely coated.
6. Place the baking dish in the preheated oven and bake for 15-
   20 minutes, or until the cod flakes easily with a fork and is
   cooked through.

7. Serve the cod filets with the tomato basil sauce spooned over the top.

Garlic Butter Shrimp

Calories per Serving:
220

Fat: 14g

Protein: 21g

Carbohydrates: 2g

Gluten-Free: Yes

Dairy-Free: No

Vegan: No

Prep Time: 10 minutes Cooking Time: 10 minutes Serving Size: 4 servings

1 lb large shrimp, peeled and deveined

3 tablespoons unsalted butter or ghee for a dairy-free option

4 cloves garlic, minced

1 tablespoon fresh lemon juice or 1 teaspoon lemon zest

1/4 teaspoon red pepper flakes

1/4 cup fresh parsley, chopped

1/2 teaspoon ground turmeric

Salt and black pepper

1. Peel and devein the shrimp if not previously done. Mince the garlic and cut the parsley.
2. In a large pan, melt the butter (or ghee) over medium heat. Add the minced garlic and sauté for 1-2 minutes, until fragrant but not browned.
3. Add the shrimp to the skillet in a single layer. Cook for 2-3 minutes on each side, until pink and opaque.
4. Once the shrimp are cooked, whisk in the lemon juice, red pepper flakes (if used), and powdered turmeric (if using). Season with salt and black pepper to taste.
5. Remove from heat and whisk in the chopped parsley.

Seafood Paella

Calories per Serving:
350

Fat: 10g

Protein: 25g

Carbohydrates: 40g

Prep Time: 20 minutes **Cooking Time:** 40 minutes **Serving Size:** 4 servings

Gluten-Free: Yes

Dairy-Free: Yes

Vegan: No

1 tablespoon olive oil

1 onion, finely chopped

3 garlic cloves, minced

1 red bell pepper, diced

1 green bell pepper, diced

1 cup diced tomatoes (canned or fresh)

1 cup short-grain brown rice (for a more traditional texture; use white rice for quicker cooking)

1 1/2 cups low-sodium vegetable broth or chicken broth

1/2 cup frozen peas

1 teaspoon smoked paprika

1/2 teaspoon ground turmeric

1/2 teaspoon ground cumin

1/4 teaspoon saffron threads

1/2 pound shrimp, peeled and deveined

1/2 pound mussels, cleaned and debearded

1/2 pound clams, cleaned

1 lemon, cut into wedges

Fresh parsley, chopped

1. Gather and prepare all the components. If using saffron, soak it in a little quantity of boiling water for 5 minutes to unleash its color and taste.
2. Heat olive oil in a large skillet or paella pan over medium heat. Add the onion and garlic, and sauté until softened, approximately 5 minutes. Add the red and green bell peppers and sauté for an additional 3 minutes.
3. Stir in the chopped tomatoes, smoked paprika, turmeric, cumin, and saffron (if using). Cook for 2 minutes until aromatic. Add the rice and toss well to coat it with the spices.
4. Pour in the veggie broth and bring to a boil. Reduce heat to low, cover, and simmer for 20 minutes. Check the rice for doneness; it should be soft but slightly firm. If required, add a little more broth or water.
5. Arrange the shrimp, mussels, and clams on top of the rice. Cover and simmer for another 10-15 minutes, until the seafood is cooked through and the mussels and clams have opened. Discard any that remain closed.
6. Garnish with fresh parsley and lemon wedges. Serve hot.

Short-Grain Brown Rice gives a heartier texture but may need slightly longer cooking time compared to white rice.

Saffron is optional but offers a real paella taste. You may eliminate it or use turmeric as a replacement for color.

Ensure seafood is fresh for the finest flavor. Frozen seafood may be utilized but should be thawed before cooking.

Turmeric Chicken and Vegetables

Calories per Serving: 300

Fat: 12g

Protein: 28g

Carbohydrates: 22g

Prep Time: 15 minutes Cooking Time: 30 minutes Serving Size: 4 servings

1 lb (450g) boneless, skinless chicken thighs, cut into bite-sized pieces

2 cups broccoli florets

1 cup diced carrots

1 cup diced sweet potatoes

1 tablespoon olive oil

Gluten-Free: Yes

1 tablespoon ground turmeric

Dairy-Free: Yes

1/2 teaspoon ground cumin

Vegan: No

1/2 teaspoon ground coriander

1/2 teaspoon paprika

1/2 teaspoon garlic powder

1/2 teaspoon onion powder

Salt and black pepper, to taste

1 lemon, juiced

1 tablespoon chopped fresh parsley

1. Cut the chicken and veggies into bite-sized pieces. Preheat the oven to 400°F (200°C).
2. In a large bowl, mix the chicken pieces with olive oil, turmeric, cumin, coriander, paprika, garlic powder, onion powder, salt, and black pepper. Mix thoroughly to coat the chicken evenly.
3. In another dish, combine the broccoli, carrots, and sweet potatoes with a little of olive oil, salt, and pepper.
4. Spread the seasoned chicken and veggies equally on a baking sheet. Place in the preheated oven and roast for 25-30 minutes, or until the chicken is cooked through and the veggies are soft. Stir halfway through for even cooking.

5. Once done, remove from the oven and sprinkle with lemon juice. Toss to blend.
6. Garnish with chopped fresh parsley if wanted and serve hot..

Ginger Beef Stir-Fry

Calories per Serving: 300

Fat: 16g

Protein: 25g

Carbohydrates: 20g

Gluten-Free: Yes

Dairy-Free: Yes

Paleo: Yes

Prep Time: 15 minutes Cooking Time: 10 minutes Serving Size: 2 servings

8 oz (225g) beef sirloin, thinly sliced

1 tablespoon fresh ginger, peeled and grated

2 cloves garlic, minced

1 tablespoon coconut oil (or olive oil)

1 bell pepper, sliced (any color)

1 cup broccoli florets

1 medium carrot, julienned

2 tablespoons gluten-free soy sauce or coconut aminos

1 tablespoon apple cider vinegar

1 tablespoon sesame seeds

1 green onion, chopped

1. Thinly slice the meat and prepare veggies. Grate the ginger and cut the garlic.
2. Heat the coconut oil in a large pan or wok over medium-high heat. Add the meat slices and simmer for 3-4 minutes, or until browned and cooked through. Remove the steak from the pan and put aside.
3. In the same skillet, add a bit of extra oil if required. Add the garlic and ginger, simmering for approximately 1 minute until fragrant. Add the bell pepper, broccoli, and carrot. Stir-fry for 4-5 minutes, or until veggies are tender-crisp.
4. Return the meat to the skillet with the veggies. Add the gluten-free soy sauce or coconut aminos and apple cider vinegar. Stir well to blend and heat for a further 1-2 minutes, letting the flavors to merge.

5. Sprinkle with sesame seeds and chopped green onion if preferred. Serve hot.

Lemon Herb Chicken

Calories per Serving:
280

Fat: 10g

Protein: 35g

Carbohydrates: 3g

Prep Time: 10 minutes Cooking Time: 25 minutes Serving Size: 4 servings

4 boneless, skinless chicken breasts

2 tablespoons olive oil

1 lemon, juiced

1 tablespoon lemon zest

2 cloves garlic, minced

1 tablespoon fresh rosemary, chopped or 1 teaspoon dried rosemary

1 tablespoon fresh thyme, chopped or 1 teaspoon dried thyme

1 teaspoon ground turmeric

1/2 teaspoon paprika

Salt and pepper

Gluten-Free: Yes

Dairy-Free: Yes

Vegan: No

1. In a bowl, add the olive oil, lemon juice, lemon zest, minced garlic, rosemary, thyme, turmeric, paprika, salt, and pepper. Mix thoroughly. Add the chicken breasts and cover them completely with the marinade. Cover and chill for at least 30 minutes (or up to 4 hours for extra flavor).
2. Preheat your oven to 400°F (200°C).
3. Remove the chicken breasts from the marinade and lay them on a baking sheet lined with parchment paper. Bake in the preheated oven for 20-25 minutes, or until the chicken is cooked through and the internal temperature reaches 165°F (74°C).
4. Let the chicken rest for 5 minutes before slicing. Serve with your choice of anti-inflammatory sides, such as steamed vegetables or a fresh salad.

Turkey and Potato Skillet

Calories per Serving: 350

Fat: 15g

Protein: 25g

Carbohydrates: 35g

Prep Time: 10 minutes Cooking Time: 25 minutes Serving Size: 4 servings

1 lb (450g) ground turkey preferably lean

2 medium sweet potatoes, peeled and diced

1 red bell pepper, chopped

1 cup chopped spinach (or kale)

1 small onion, diced

2 cloves garlic, minced

1 tablespoon olive oil

1 teaspoon ground turmeric

1/2 teaspoon ground cumin

1/2 teaspoon smoked paprika

Salt and pepper

Fresh parsley or cilantro

Gluten-Free: Yes

Dairy-Free: Yes

Vegan: No

1. **Gather All Necessary Ingredients:** Peel and dice the sweet potatoes, cut the bell pepper, and dice the onion. Mince the garlic.
2. **Heat olive oil in a large pan over medium heat. Add the chopped onion and sauté until transparent, approximately 3 minutes. Add the minced garlic and simmer for another minute until fragrant. Add the ground turkey, breaking it up with a spoon, and heat until browned and well cooked through, approximately 7-10 minutes. Remove the cooked turkey from the pan and put aside.**
3. **In the same skillet, add a bit of extra olive oil if required. Add the diced sweet potatoes and simmer, turning regularly, until they begin to soften, approximately 10 minutes.**
4. **Return the cooked turkey to the skillet with the sweet potatoes. Add the diced bell pepper, spinach, turmeric, cumin, smoked paprika, salt, and pepper. Stir well to mix and simmer for another 5-7 minutes, until the sweet potatoes are cooked and the spinach has wilted.**
5. **Garnish with fresh parsley or cilantro if preferred. Serve hot.**

Rosemary Garlic Lamb Chops

Calories per Serving: 50

Fat: 24g

Protein: 30g

Carbohydrates: 2g

Prep Time: 15 minutes Cooking Time: 15 minutes Serving Size: 2 servings (2 lamb chops each)

4 lamb chops about 1 inch thick

2 tablespoons fresh rosemary, finely chopped or 1 tablespoon dried rosemary

4 cloves garlic, minced

2 tablespoons extra virgin olive oil

1 teaspoon sea salt

1/2 teaspoon black pepper

1 teaspoon lemon juice

1/2 teaspoon paprika

Gluten-Free: Yes

Dairy-Free: Yes

Paleo: Yes

1. In a small bowl, mix the rosemary, garlic, olive oil, sea salt, black pepper, and lemon juice (if using). Mix thoroughly.
2. Rub the mixture all over the lamb chops, ensuring they are uniformly covered. Let the lamb chops marinate at room temperature for 15-30 minutes, or refrigerate for up to 2 hours if prepared ahead.
3. Preheat a grill or a skillet over medium-high heat. If using a skillet, you may need to add a little additional olive oil to avoid sticking.
4. Place the lamb chops on the grill or skillet. Cook for 4-5 minutes on each side for medium-rare, or longer if you want them more done. Use a meat thermometer to check for doneness: 145°F (63°C) for medium-rare.
5. Remove the lamb chops from the pan and let them rest for 5 minutes before serving. This helps the liquids redistribute and keeps the meat tender.

CHAPTER 9

SMALL BITES, DIPS AND SPREADS

Turmeric Roasted Chickpeas

Sweet Potato Bites

Cucumber Hummus Bites

Carrot and Ginger Energy Balls

Avocado Cilantro Dip

Spicy Black Bean Dip

Roasted Red Pepper Dip

Pumpkin Seed Pesto

Cucumber Mint Yogurt Dip

Sweet Potato Hummus

Turmeric Roasted Chickpeas

Calories per Serving:
180

Prep Time: 10 minutes Cooking Time: 25-30 minutes Serving Size: 1 cup

Fat: 5g

Protein: 7g

Carbohydrates: 24g

1 can (15 oz) chickpeas, drained and rinsed	**1/2 teaspoon garlic powder**
1 tablespoon olive oil	**1/4 teaspoon ground black pepper**
1 teaspoon ground turmeric	**1/4 teaspoon sea salt**
1/2 teaspoon ground cumin	
1/2 teaspoon smoked paprika	

Gluten-Free: Yes

Dairy-Free: Yes

Vegan: Yes

Nut-Free: Yes

1. Preheat your oven to 400°F (200°C). Line a baking sheet with parchment paper for easy cleaning.
2. After draining and washing the chickpeas, blot them dry completely with a paper towel. This step is vital for getting crispy chickpeas.
3. In a large bowl, stir the dry chickpeas with olive oil, turmeric, cumin, smoked paprika, garlic powder, black pepper, and sea salt until equally covered.
4. Spread the seasoned chickpeas in a single layer on the prepared baking sheet. Roast in the preheated oven for 25-30 minutes, stirring the pan halfway through, until the chickpeas are golden and crispy.
5. Allow the roasted chickpeas to cool fully on the baking sheet before serving. They will continue to crisp up as they cool.
6. Make sure chickpeas are thoroughly covered with oil and spices for even taste and crispiness.

7. Store leftover roasted chickpeas in an airtight jar at room temperature for up to a week. They may lose some crispiness over time, so consume them fresh for the best texture.
8. Feel free to modify the spices according to your taste. Adding a sprinkle of cayenne pepper might give them an additional kick.

Sweet Potato Bites

Calories per Serving: 150

Fat: 5g

Protein: 2g

Carbohydrates: 25g

Prep Time: 15 minutes Cooking Time: 25 minutes Serving Size: 4 servings (4-5 bites per serving)

2 medium sweet potatoes, peeled and cut into 1-inch cubes

1 tablespoon olive oil

1/2 teaspoon ground turmeric

1/2 teaspoon paprika

1/2 teaspoon ground cumin

1/4 teaspoon garlic powder

1/4 teaspoon onion powder

Salt and black pepper

Fresh parsley or cilantro, chopped

Gluten-Free: Yes

Dairy-Free: Yes

Vegan: Yes

1. Preheat your oven to 400°F (200°C) and line a baking sheet with parchment paper.
2. In a large bowl, mix the sweet potato cubes with olive oil, turmeric, paprika, cumin, garlic powder, onion powder, salt, and black pepper until equally coated.
3. Spread the seasoned sweet potato cubes in a single layer on the prepared baking sheet. Bake for 20-25 minutes, or until the sweet potatoes are soft and slightly crispy on the edges. Shake the pan or stir the cubes halfway through cooking for even roasting
4. Remove from the oven and let cool slightly. Garnish with chopped parsley or cilantro if preferred. Serve warm as a snack or side dish..

Cucumber Hummus Bites

Calories per Serving:
120

Fat: 6g

Protein: 4g

Carbohydrates: 14g

Prep Time: 10 minutes Serving Size: 4 servings (8-10 bites per serving)

1 large cucumber, sliced into rounds about 1/4 inch thick

1 cup hummus store-bought or homemade, ensure it's made without dairy or gluten

1 tablespoon extra-virgin olive oil

1/2 teaspoon ground cumin

1/4 teaspoon smoked paprika

Fresh parsley or cilantro, chopped

Sea salt and black pepper

Gluten-Free: Yes

Dairy-Free: Yes

Vegan: Yes

Nut-Free: Yes

1. Wash and slice the cucumber into rounds. Pat them dry with a paper towel to ensure they're not too wet.
2. If desired, combine the hummus with ground cumin and smoked paprika for added flavor. Adjust seasoning with sea salt and black pepper.
3. Spoon a tiny dollop of hummus onto each cucumber slice.
4. Drizzle a little extra-virgin olive oil over the top of each mouthful. Garnish with chopped parsley or cilantro.
5. Arrange the cucumber hummus bits on a plate

Carrot and Ginger Energy Balls

Calories per Serving: 90

Fat: 4g

Protein: 2g

Carbohydrates: 11g

Prep Time: 15 minutes Serving Size: 12 balls (1 ball per serving)

Gluten-Free: Yes

Dairy-Free: Yes

Vegan: Yes

Nut-Free: No

1 cup finely shredded carrots (about 2 medium carrots)

1/2 cup rolled oats (gluten-free if needed)

1/2 cup unsweetened shredded coconut

1/4 cup chopped nuts, almonds or walnuts or seeds like sunflower seeds for a nut-free option

1/4 cup almond butter or sunflower seed butter for a nut-free version

2 tablespoons honey or maple syrup

1 tablespoon ground ginger or 1 tablespoon freshly grated ginger

1/2 teaspoon ground cinnamon

A pinch of salt

1. Grate the carrots and cut the nuts if required.
2. In a large bowl, mix the shredded carrots, rolled oats, shredded coconut, chopped nuts or seeds, almond butter, honey or maple syrup, ground ginger, ground cinnamon, and a sprinkle of salt. Mix thoroughly until everything is uniformly distributed.
3. Use your hands or a tiny cookie scoop to mold the dough into bite-sized balls, approximately 1 inch in diameter. If the mixture is too dry, add a bit more almond butter or honey.
4. Place the balls on a parchment-lined baking sheet or dish. Chill in the refrigerator for at least 30 minutes to firm up.
5. Store the energy balls in an airtight jar in the fridge for up to a week.

Avocado Cilantro Dip

Calories per Serving: 90

Fat: 8g

Prep Time: 10 minutes Serving Size: 1/4 cup

Protein: 1g

Carbohydrates: 5g

2 ripe avocados, peeled and pitted

1/2 cup fresh cilantro leaves

1 small garlic clove, minced

1 tablespoon lime juice about 1/2 lime

1/4 teaspoon ground cumin

1/4 teaspoon sea salt or to taste

1/4 teaspoon ground black pepper (optional)

1 small jalapeño, seeded and chopped

Gluten-Free: Yes

Dairy-Free: Yes

Vegan: Yes

Nut-Free: Yes

1. Cut the avocados in halves, remove the pits, and scoop the flesh into a food processor or blender. If using fresh jalapeño, cut it finely and keep away.
2. Add the cilantro leaves, minced garlic, lime juice, ground cumin, and sea salt to the food processor. If using, add the black pepper and jalapeño.
3. Blend until the mixture is smooth and creamy. You may need to scrape along the edges of the processor to ensure everything is properly blended.
4. Taste the dip and adjust the seasoning with extra salt or lime juice as required.
5. Transfer the dip to a dish and serve or chill in the refrigerator until ready to use.

Spicy Black Bean Dip

Calories per Serving: 130

Fat: 2g

Protein: 6g

Carbohydrates: 22g

Prep Time: 10 minutes Serving Size: 1/2 cup (makes about 4 servings)

1 can (15 oz) black beans, drained and rinsed

1 tablespoon extra virgin olive oil

1/2 cup diced tomatoes (fresh or canned)

1/4 cup finely chopped red onion

1 small jalapeño, seeded and minced

2 cloves garlic, minced

1 teaspoon ground cumin

1/2 teaspoon smoked paprika

1/2 teaspoon ground turmeric

Juice of 1 lime

Salt and black pepper

2 tablespoons chopped fresh cilantro

Gluten-Free: Yes

Dairy-Free: Yes

Vegan: Yes

Nut-Free: Yes

1. Ensure the black beans are drained and washed properly. If using fresh tomatoes, dice them thinly.
2. In a mixing dish, combine the black beans, diced tomatoes, red onion, minced jalapeño, minced garlic, ground cumin, smoked paprika, and turmeric (if using). Mix thoroughly.
3. Add the olive oil, lime juice, salt, and black pepper. Stir to blend fully.
4. For a smoother texture, you may partly mash the beans with a fork or use a potato masher. If you like a chunky dip, stir until thoroughly blended without mashing.

5. Transfer to a serving dish and garnish with chopped cilantro if desired. Serve immediately with vegetable sticks or gluten-free crackers.

The heat from the jalapeño might vary. Start with a tiny quantity and taste as you go.

The dip may be kept in an airtight jar in the refrigerator for up to 3 days.

Roasted Red Pepper Dip

Calories per Serving: 80

Fat: 6g

Protein: 2g

Carbohydrates: 6g

Prep Time: 10 minutes Cooking Time: 25 minutes Serving Size: 1/4 cup

2 large red bell peppers	1/4 teaspoon ground cumin
1 tablespoon olive oil	1/4 teaspoon smoked paprika
1 small garlic clove, minced	Salt and pepper
1 tablespoon lemon juice	1 tablespoon fresh parsley or basil

Gluten-Free: Yes

Dairy-Free: Yes

Vegan: Yes

Nut-Free: Yes

1. Preheat the oven to 425°F (220°C). Place the red bell peppers on a baking sheet and roast for 20-25 minutes, turning regularly, until the skins are blackened and blistered.
2. Remove the peppers from the oven and set them in a dish covered with plastic wrap or a kitchen towel. Let them steam for 10 minutes to make peeling simpler. Peel off the skins, remove the stems and seeds, and coarsely cut the meat.
3. In a food processor or high-speed blender, mix the roasted red peppers, olive oil, minced garlic, lemon juice, ground cumin, smoked paprika, salt, and pepper. Blend until smooth.
4. Transfer the dip to a bowl and garnish with chopped parsley or basil if desired. Serve with veggie sticks or gluten-free crackers.

Pumpkin Seed Pesto

Calories per Serving:
180

Fat: 16g

Protein: 7g

Carbohydrates: 5g

Prep Time: 10 minutes Serving Size: 1/4 cup

1 cup raw pumpkin seeds (pepitas)

1 cup fresh basil leaves (packed)

1/2 cup fresh parsley leaves (packed)

1/4 cup extra-virgin olive oil

2 cloves garlic, peeled

2 tablespoons nutritional yeast

1 tablespoon lemon juice

1/4 teaspoon sea salt

1/4 teaspoon black pepper

Gluten-Free: Yes

Dairy-Free: Yes

Vegan: Yes

Nut-Free: Yes

1. For a richer flavor, gently toast the pumpkin seeds in a dry pan over medium heat for 2-3 minutes, tossing regularly. Allow to cool.
2. In a food processor or high-speed blender, mix the raw or roasted pumpkin seeds, basil, parsley, garlic, nutritional yeast (if using), lemon juice, sea salt, and black pepper.
3. With the processor running, carefully trickle in the olive oil until the mixture achieves a smooth, creamy consistency. You may need to pause and scrape down the sides periodically.
4. Taste the pesto and adjust the seasoning as required. Add additional salt, pepper, or lemon juice to suit your liking.
5. Transfer the pesto to a jar or airtight container. It may be used immediately or kept in the refrigerator for up to one week.
6. To keep freshness, coat the surface of the pesto with a thin layer of olive oil before closing the container.

Cucumber Mint Yogurt Dip

Calories per Serving:
120

Fat: 6g

Protein: 6g

Carbohydrates: 10g

Prep Time: 10 minutes Serving Size: 1 cup

1 cup plain Greek yogurt

1 medium cucumber, peeled, seeded, and finely diced

2 tablespoons fresh mint leaves, chopped

1 tablespoon fresh lemon juice

1 clove garlic, minced

1/2 teaspoon ground turmeric

Salt and pepper

Gluten-Free: Yes

Dairy-Free: No

Vegan: No

Nut-Free: Yes

1. Peel and seed the cucumber, then finely cut it. Chop the mint leaves and mince the garlic.
2. In a mixing dish, combine the Greek yogurt, sliced cucumber, chopped mint, lemon juice, and minced garlic. If using, add the ground turmeric.
3. Stir everything together until fully incorporated. Season with salt and pepper to taste.
4. For the finest taste, let the dip rest in the refrigerator for at least 30 minutes to enable the flavors to mingle.
5. Serve chilled as a dip with fresh veggies, whole grain crackers, or as a topping for salads.

Substitute Greek yogurt with a dairy-free yogurt prepared from coconut, almond, or cashew milk.

Sweet Potato Hummus

Calories per Serving: 90

Fat: 4g

Prep Time: 10 minutes Cooking Time: 25 minutes Serving Size: 1/4 cup

Protein: 3g

Carbohydrates: 13g

1 medium sweet potato about 1 cup, peeled and cubed

1 can (15 oz) chickpeas, drained and rinsed

1/4 cup tahini (sesame paste)

2 tablespoons olive oil

1 tablespoon lemon juice

1 garlic clove, minced

1/2 teaspoon ground cumin

1/2 teaspoon smoked paprika

1/4 teaspoon ground turmeric

Salt and pepper

Gluten-Free: Yes

Dairy-Free: Yes

Vegan: Yes

Nut-Free: Yes

1. Preheat the oven to 400°F (200°C). Place the sweet potato cubes on a baking sheet, sprinkle with a little olive oil, and season with salt and pepper. Roast for 20-25 minutes, or until soft and faintly caramelized. Allow to cool slightly.

2. In a food processor, mix the roasted sweet potato, chickpeas, tahini, olive oil, lemon juice, minced garlic, cumin, smoked paprika, and turmeric (if using). Blend until smooth and creamy, scraping down the sides as required. Adjust seasoning with salt and pepper to taste.

3. Transfer the hummus to a bowl. Serve with fresh veggies, whole-grain crackers, or as a spread in wraps and sandwiches.

APPENDICES

30 DAYS MEAL PLAN

First Week

Day 1
- Breakfast: Berry Banana Smoothie
- Lunch: Turmeric Chickpea Salad
- Dinner: Turmeric Chicken Soup
- Snack: Turmeric Roasted Chickpeas

Day 2
- Breakfast: Mango Ginger Smoothie
- Lunch: Chickpea Salad Sandwich
- Dinner: Garlic Butter Shrimp
- Snack: Sweet Potato Bites

Day 3
- Breakfast: Turmeric Pineapple Smoothie
- Lunch: Black Bean and Quinoa Wrap
- Dinner: Spinach and Sweet Potato Frittata
- Snack: Cucumber Hummus Bites

Day 4

- Breakfast: Apple Spinach Smoothie
- Lunch: Barley and Mushroom Risotto
- Dinner: Mackerel with Lemon
- Snack: Carrot and Ginger Energy Balls

Day 5

- Breakfast: Beetroot Berry Smoothie
- Lunch: Avocado and Egg Sandwich
- Dinner: Sweet Potato and Spinach Skillet
- Snack: Spicy Black Bean Dip

Day 6

- Breakfast: Cherry Almond Smoothie
- Lunch: Beet and Arugula Salad
- Dinner: Quinoa and Sweet Potato Chili
- Snack: Roasted Red Pepper Dip

Day 7

- Breakfast: Citrus Carrot Smoothie
- Lunch: Brown Rice and Bean Burrito
- Dinner: Ginger Beef Stir-Fry
- Snack: Pumpkin Seed Pesto

Second Week 2

Day 8

- Breakfast: Blueberry Avocado Smoothie
- Lunch: Black Bean and Corn Salad
- Dinner: Lentil and Spinach Soup
- Snack: Cucumber Mint Yogurt Dip

Day 9

- Breakfast: Green Smoothie
- Lunch: Falafel Wrap

- Dinner: Cod with Tomato Basil Sauce
- Snack: Sweet Potato Hummus

Day 10
- Breakfast: Strawberry Basil Smoothie
- Lunch: Apple Walnut Salad
- Dinner: Mushroom and Barley Soup
- Snack: Sweet Potato Bites

Day 11
- Breakfast: Ginger Peach Smoothie
- Lunch: Quinoa and Black Bean Tacos
- Dinner: Turkey and Potato Skillet
- Snack: Avocado Cilantro Dip

Day 12
- Breakfast: Cucumber Mint Smoothie
- Lunch: Millet and Vegetable Stir-Fry
- Dinner: Kale and White Bean Soup
- Snack: Spicy Chickpea Stew

Day 13
- Breakfast: Papaya Turmeric Smoothie
- Lunch: Chicken and Spinach Wrap
- Dinner: Seafood Paella
- Snack: Roasted Red Pepper Dip

Day 14
- Breakfast: Raspberry Chia Smoothie
- Lunch: Bulgur Wheat and Chickpea Salad
- Dinner: Turmeric Shrimp Stir-Fry
- Snack: Turmeric Roasted Chickpeas

Third Week

Day 15
- Breakfast: Pomegranate Beet Smoothie
- Lunch: Wild Rice and Cranberry Salad
- Dinner: Broccoli and Spinach Soup
- Snack: Carrot and Ginger Energy Balls

Day 16
- Breakfast: Kiwi Spinach Smoothie
- Lunch: Black Bean and Quinoa Wrap
- Dinner: Lemon Herb Chicken
- Snack: Sweet Potato Hummus

Day 17
- Breakfast: Orange Carrot Smoothie
- Lunch: Beet and Arugula Salad
- Dinner: Pea and Mint Soup
- Snack: Cucumber Hummus Bites

Day 18
- Breakfast: Watermelon Mint Smoothie
- Lunch: Chickpea and Spinach Curry
- Dinner: Rosemary Garlic Lamb Chops
- Snack: Spicy Black Bean Dip

Day 19
- Breakfast: Apple Cinnamon Smoothie
- Lunch: Quinoa Vegetable Soup
- Dinner: Egg and Sweet Potato Casserole
- Snack: Pumpkin Seed Pesto

Day 20
- Breakfast: Turmeric Banana Pancakes
- Lunch: Chicken and Spinach Wrap

- Dinner: Miso Soup with Tofu
- Snack: Roasted Red Pepper Dip

Day 21
- Breakfast: Gingerbread Pancakes
- Lunch: Falafel Wrap
- Dinner: Cod with Tomato Basil Sauce
- Snack: Avocado Cilantro Dip

Week 4

Day 22
- Breakfast: Pumpkin Spice Pancakes
- Lunch: Black Bean and Corn Salad
- Dinner: Quinoa and Sweet Potato Chili
- Snack: Turmeric Roasted Chickpeas

Day 23
- Breakfast: Matcha Green Tea Pancakes
- Lunch: Turmeric Chickpea Salad
- Dinner: Kale and White Bean Soup
- Snack: Sweet Potato Bites

Day 24
- Breakfast: Lemon Poppy Seed Pancakes
- Lunch: Wild Rice and Cranberry Salad
- Dinner: Garlic Butter Shrimp
- Snack: Cucumber Mint Yogurt Dip

Day 25
- Breakfast: Beetroot Pancakes
- Lunch: Apple Walnut Salad
- Dinner: Mushroom and Barley Soup
- Snack: Carrot and Ginger Energy Balls

Day 26
- Breakfast: Coconut Flour Waffles
- Lunch: Black Bean and Quinoa Wrap
- Dinner: Broccoli and Spinach Soup
- Snack: Sweet Potato Hummus

Day 27
- Breakfast: Buckwheat Waffles
- Lunch: Quinoa and Black Bean Tacos
- Dinner: Ginger Beef Stir-Fry
- Snack: Pumpkin Seed Pesto

Day 28
- Breakfast: Flaxseed Waffles
- Lunch: Chickpea and Spinach Curry
- Dinner: Baked Eggs in Potato Nests
- Snack: Avocado Cilantro Dip

Day 29
- Breakfast: Turmeric Waffles
- Lunch: Bulgur Wheat and Chickpea Salad
- Dinner: Turmeric Chicken and Vegetables
- Snack: Roasted Red Pepper Dip

Day 30
- Breakfast: Sweet Potato Waffles
- Lunch: Berry Spinach Salad
- Dinner: Mackerel with Lemon
- Snack: Spicy Black Bean Dip

REFERENCES

Dobaczewski, M., Xia, Y., Bujak, M., Gonzalez-Quesada, C., & Frangogiannis, N. G. (2010). CCR5 signaling suppresses inflammation and reduces adverse remodeling of the infarcted heart, mediating recruitment of regulatory T cells. American Journal of Pathology, 176(5), 2177–2187. https://doi.org/10.2353/ajpath.2010.090759

Kaluza, J., Håkansson, N., Harris, H. R., Orsini, N., Michaëlsson, K., & Wolk, A. (2018). Influence of anti-inflammatory diet and smoking on mortality and survival in men and women: two prospective cohort studies. Journal of Internal Medicine, 285(1), 75–91. https://doi.org/10.1111/joim.12823

Marcason, W. (2010). What is the Anti-Inflammatory diet? Journal of the American Dietetic Association, 110(11), 1780. https://doi.org/10.1016/j.jada.2010.09.024

Olendzki, B. C., Silverstein, T. D., Persuitte, G. M., Ma, Y., Baldwin, K. R., & Cave, D. (2014). An anti-inflammatory diet as treatment for inflammatory bowel disease: a case series report. Nutrition Journal, 13(1). https://doi.org/10.1186/1475-2891-13-5

Quévrain, E., Maubert, M., Michon, C., Chain, F., Marquant, R., Tailhades, J., Miquel, S., Carlier, L., Bermúdez-Humarán, L., Pigneur, B., Lequin, O., Kharrat, P., Thomas, G., Rainteau, D., Aubry, C., Breyner, N., Afonso, C., Lavielle, S., Grill, J., . . . Seksik, P. (2015). Identification of an anti-inflammatory protein fromFaecalibacterium prausnitzii, a commensal bacterium deficient in Crohn's disease. Gut, 65(3), 415–425. https://doi.org/10.1136/gutjnl-2014-307649

Sears, B. (2015). Anti-inflammatory diets. Journal of the American College of Nutrition, 34(sup1), 14–21. https://doi.org/10.1080/07315724.2015.1080105

Tedelind, S., Westberg, F., Kjerrulf, M., & Vidal, A. (2007). Anti-inflammatory properties of the short-chain fatty acids acetate and propionate: A study with relevance to inflammatory bowel disease. World Journal of Gastroenterology, 13(20), 2826. https://doi.org/10.3748/wjg.v13.i20.2826

Vadell, A. K., Bärebring, L., Hulander, E., Gjertsson, I., Lindqvist, H. M., & Winkvist, A. (2020). Anti-inflammatory Diet In Rheumatoid Arthritis (ADIRA)—a randomized, controlled crossover trial indicating effects on disease activity. American Journal of Clinical Nutrition, 111(6), 1203–1213. https://doi.org/10.1093/ajcn/nqaa019

Woelber, J. P., Gärtner, M., Breuninger, L., Anderson, A., König, D., Hellwig, E., Al-Ahmad, A., Vach, K., Dötsch, A., Ratka-Krüger, P., & Tennert, C. (2019). The influence of an anti-inflammatory diet on gingivitis. A randomized controlled trial. Journal of Clinical Periodontology, 46(4), 481–490. https://doi.org/10.1111/jcpe.13094

Yan, Q., Zhang, J., Liu, H., Babu-Khan, S., Vassar, R., Biere, A. L., Citron, M., & Landreth, G. (2003). Anti-Inflammatory drug therapy alters B-Amyloid processing and deposition in an animal model of Alzheimer's disease. Journal of Neuroscience, 23(20), 7504–7509. https://doi.org/10.1523/jneurosci.23-20-07504.2003

Scheiber, A., & Mank, V. (2023, October 28). Anti-Inflammatory diets. StatPearls - NCBI Bookshelf. https://www.ncbi.nlm.nih.gov/books/NBK597377/

RECIPE INDEX

Made in the USA
Las Vegas, NV
11 October 2024